Patient Better

The Remote Companion for Self-Health Management

Jennifer Woodruff, MHA

Patient Better: The Remote Companion for Self-Health Management

Written By:

Jennifer Woodruff, MHA

Copyright © 2021

Patient Better LLC

ISBN 13: 978-0-578678160

Library of Congress Control Number: 2020906789

For Information and bulk ordering, contact:

Patient Better LLC

Toll-Free: 1 (866) 205-2309

orders@PatientBetter.com

Disclaimer

All content found on the PatientBetter.com Website, handbooks, workbooks, including text, images, audio, or other formats, were created for informational purposes only. The content is not intended to be a substitute for professional medical advice, diagnosis, or treatment.

Always seek the advice of your licensed health care professional with any questions that you may have regarding a medical condition. Never disregard professional medical advice or delay in seeking it because of something that you have read in the realm of Patient Better's reading material. If you think that you may have a medical emergency, call your practitioner, go to the emergency department, or call 911 immediately.

Patient Better does not recommend or endorse any specific tests, physicians, products, procedures, opinions, or other information that may be on Patient Better's handbook or website Reliance on any information provided by Patient Better handbook, PatientBetter.com, contracted representatives, writers, or medical professionals presenting content for publication to Patient Better is solely at your own risk. All information found on PatientBetter.com Website and Handbook was believed to be correct at the time of inclusion, and it is for informational purposes only and not intended as medical advice. References to any treatment or therapy option or to any program, treatment, or service do not constitute official endorsement by Patient Better, Readers are encouraged to fully investigate treatment options and providers that may be more appropriate for specific medical treatment.

The Patient Better *Self-Managing* Program

The Patient Better program is a curriculum that helps people learn about the healthcare industry and ultimately become proficient in self-managing care. This program specializes in helping patients and their family-member caregivers to form an at-home care team, enhance communication with health professionals, and organize care through a personal, medical managing system.

Whether your goal is to take better care of yourself, enhance your capabilities of how to care for others, or provide long-distance care for a loved one, this is the one program that can help you develop and refine your caregiving potential. Patient Better helps people to better manage care through *meaningful learning*.

Meaningful learning is a universally recognized concept where people apply previously learned information and connect it to the newly acquired information. Many of Patient Better's students come from diverse backgrounds. And so, we begin training at the grassroots of this industry by defining healthcare administration principles. And depending on your familiarity with the healthcare industry, you will have a starting point where you can begin to tackle different situations that may arise.

Upon reading this book, not only will you have a beginning point of where to start training about care, you will have the in-depth knowledge of how to take better care of your health and enhance your caregiving proficiency to take care of someone else. This book is your starting point to take self-managing care to the next level and have a better vision to know what to do to stay current on the latest technologies that are being used in the industry to conduct a proper telemedicine appointment.

Furthermore, you will learn what is needed to be done as a patient to have an equal partnership with providers, to engage in a productive in-person and virtual medical appointment, and traverse through the two when appropriate.

Patient Better supplies people with the following benefits

Enhanced Participation in Treatment – Patients have fewer complications, fewer visits to emergency rooms, are prepared for an information-driven medical appointment while reducing unforeseen costs.

When we are responsible for the health management of our family members. Or when patients have to rely on others to provide assistance for documentation, medication, and activities for daily living. If not done correctly, this might put a severe strain not only on the patient but also on the caregiver. Knowing about the patient, their diagnosis, treatments, and their medications can give the caregivers and the patients peace of mind, deliver more quality care, allows everyone involved to focus on more instrumental tasks-like getting back to health. Today, it has become an invaluable help for the patient to have an additional at-home caregiver to be involved in the professional's and patient's conversation. Not only does it provide an enormous amount of comfort but an additional at-home caregiver is able to help in decision making. In instances like this, the Self-Health Manager is the ideal communicator while remaining compliant in many situations.

Responsible Medical Utilization – Prepare for medical appointments, reduce unnecessary phone calls and office visits, and effectively take advantage of offered services, treatments, and resources.

As a patient or at-home caregiver, it is imperative that you are aware of all the resources available to you. But you won't be able to do that without the proper and up to date knowledge. By following the Patient Better program, you can count on always being prepared for medical appointments and position yourself to have fewer unnecessary phone calls and office visits. And you will also be able to effectively take advantage of the most closely matched services, treatments, and resources offered online or in your area.

Improved Risk Management – Patients have a realistic calculation of services that are required for correct treatment and recovery to make more informed healthcare choices and decisions.

Often, panic and impetuous decisions are the culprits for worsening unforeseen situations. When under pressure there is a tendency to increase the risk of difficulty and ability to decipher the needed or unnecessary care. Patient Better will help you develop an informed calculation of services and realistic projections that you need for your proper treatment and recovery. By improving your ability to manage risk, you make more conscious decisions about your care. As a result, you safeguard yourself and your family from being at risk for uncalculated compromises in treatment.

Proper Self-Management of Records – Patients become efficient collaborators in the transfer of information from one doctor's office to the next.

Having a condition, illness, or disease often requires you to pay a number of visits to specialists and ancillary care service providers in addition to your primary care physician. This will make medical record management more complex for you. It might not seem like a herculean task at first, but if you take into account collecting all the data from every healthcare providing facility and managing it, you can see the problem quite clearly. As a consequence, your documents may not be uniform across all recording databases which may make receiving care more predisposed to misinformation and errors Furthermore, some medical records from other clinics may contain valuable and pertinent information that links to your new health concern. And it may be tough to retrieve those documents. Through Patient Better, not only do you have a designated place for each document, you become an efficient collaborator and liaison to uniformly transfer information from one healthcare provider's office to the other. In this way, you are proactively protecting yourself from any important information from being lost in your medical history.

The Three Levels of Education in the Patient Better Program

The Patient Better program has three prominent levels designed to cater to your individual and specific needs. You can begin learning from any one of the following levels that are compatible with your prior industry experience.

(Level One) Beginner: Level One offers two educational tools in its arsenal: (1) the Patient Better academy and (2) the textbook. These level one items are created for people who are completely new to the world of self-managing. The "Beginner" level focuses on essential education to learn the basics and build a solid foundation for the person so they may have sufficient knowledge of the healthcare industry.

However, the beginner level is not just for those who are recently diagnosed, but also for people who want to take a more pro-active approach and begin recording for themselves or for someone they care for. By learning the fundamentals of the healthcare industry, you will be able to self-manage several conditions. People usually start to self-manage care for these mild forms of health conditions: (pre) diabetes, arthritis, or high blood pressure.

(Level Two) Intermediate: The Patient Better Workbook is the second level of self-management training. This workbook is the "hands-on" instruction for patients and caregivers who are responsible for more sophisticated at-home care delivery tasks. The intermediate level is for people with more intricate conditions and those who find it necessary to organize an at-home care team. These are the folks who are expected to meet the higher level of commitment that the proper management of complex conditions demands. The most common conditions that may involve Patient Better's level two training include Cancer, Parkinson's, dementia/Alzheimer's disease, heart failure, or any other major illness or injury.

(Level Three) Advanced: This level helps people with both level one and level two conditions to self-manage care for both in-person and virtual medical appointments. Level Three focuses on the skills that are needed for telemedicine and for the management of complex and sophisticated conditions as well as providing in-depth, at-home team management training.

The Patient Better Program

Designed for people who have experience of living in a condition where they need constant care and governance to manage their health.

Level One Tools for Newcomers

Academy

The Patient Better Academy offers a full online classroom experience with supporting course work that includes video tutorials, presentations, quizzes, and certificates. You will feel like you're back in school, but it will be worth it! This learning center is designed to provide learning even an 8th grader will be able to retain easily. Therefore, it enables many people to become more proficient within the current healthcare arena - no matter what their current level of healthcare knowledge is.

Textbook

Patient Better: A Comprehensive Guide to Self-Health Management is an instructional piece written to accommodate the primary level of self-managed care. This handbook walks people through the healthcare industry, and it is an essential tool for patients in need of a recollection tool.

Level Two Tools for the Intermediate:

Workbook

The Patient Better Workbook: Self Manage Your Way to Better Care is a collection of our most popular worksheets. These templates assist laypeople and their *informal caregivers* to further develop analytical skills and improve their ability to coordinate care.

This workbook helps patients and their informal caregivers to perform high-level administrative tasks that are part of personal healthcare management. Today, individuals with complex medical conditions (and the folks who care for them) are often required to perform sophisticated, in-home medical care. With that being said, it's more critical than ever that these tasks are properly recorded. Patient Better assists patients and their caregivers, adult children, parents, and guardians alike to keep a good document trail and to continue to collaborate care through worksheets

Level Three Tools for the Advanced

Handbook

Patient Better: The Remote Companion for Self-Health Management is an instructional guide for everyday people and their *informal caregivers* on how to organize and properly record care for both in-person and virtual medical office visits.

This book is the third and final step to our self-managing program. It is written for the independent analyst who feels ready to shoulder the responsibilities of self-care for themselves or for a loved one for both face-to-face and remote care appointments. This hybrid of self-maintenance is designed specifically to better maintain complexities in long-term conditions. And to transition the traditional provider-patient relationship into an equal partnership in care, or EPIC relationship.

Before reading this book, Patient Better recommends that you are familiar with the basic concepts of our self-managing program:

- ✓ Clearinghouse
- ✓ Informal caregiver
- ✓ The Self-Health Manager™
- ✓ Patient Better's SOAP Note, Treatment Plan Calculator & Contributor Cover Page
- ✓ The difference between standard and non-standard medical documents and records
- ✓ Healthcare outcomes and measurements
- ✓ An essential foundation of patient communication and literacy

The EPIC Relationship

The EPIC relationship can equalize your partnership with the physician. The EPIC Relationship is the starting point to sustain and grow and meet the needs of today's basic patient functionalities. Patients as Partners is a popular concept where healthcare professionals consider their patients as a full-fledged partner of their healthcare and this is where the patient's knowledge and experience are recognized. This book helps you with your transition from in-person encounters with health advisors and to a time where telemedicine consultations become the norm. Through this final step of self-managing care, you will know how to develop EPIC relationships- right from the very start.

This is the last step in the Patient Better self-management program, its elements, and the optimal destination of what your learning should look like:

1. Capable– You will have a solid foundation that will allow you to confidently self-manage care. You will be comfortable and confident in conveying and communicating health information to others (professionals, family members, and other caregivers) involved in your care.

2. Knowledgeable – When you become knowledgeable about the healthcare industry, not only will you gain pertinent knowledge regarding conditions, medications, and treatments, you will also open yourself up to a world that will stay with you throughout your entire life.

3. Understanding – You will gain a complete grasp of health communication and literacy and how proficiency impacts your care. You will be able to understand the healthcare professional's backgrounds and match their characteristics to your needs that are important to you when receiving care. Ultimately this will give you a better experience and outlook throughout your occurrence.

Preface

You may be a beginner in the healthcare world, but if your parent or grandparent or someone you deeply love is suffering from a condition that requires at-home care, you roll up your sleeves and help out, whether you know how to or not. Your love makes you want to help them, whether you are prepared or trained to care for them or not.

Indeed, with the proper education for self-management, you can acquire the knowledge you need to manage care for yourself and your loved ones. And with the right education, you will be able to help and care for them in an improved manner; you will better understand what they're going through and how you can assure them in this difficult time. You will learn how to make their lives as comfortable as possible.

Patient Better will be with you every step of the way so you can better care for yourself or bring out your full potential to deliver care to your loved ones.

After a night in the hospital, and just when you get your discharge orders, the nurse rushes into your room and provides you with a summary of your stay and a detailed list of instructions that you are expected to follow after you leave. You sigh heavily at the sight of the list and wonder, "Isn't this too much? I'm a little overwhelmed and a little unprepared for all this."

You convince yourself that you'll have better clarity when you re-read the report more thoroughly after you get home and in a clearer state of mind. So you nod your head in agreement and assure the nurse that you understand the doctor's directions. And when you finally leave the clinic, your hope is to get your life back to the way it was before you fell ill. However, with a list of self-care instructions like the one you just received; you may find that difficult to do.

After you get settled in at home, you review the doctor's directions once again and realize there is still a long way to go before things can go back to normal. Reflecting upon your stay and recalling the efficiency of the healthcare professionals and realizing how straightforward their guidance was... you wonder if you're really up to this task of recovering on your own. And thinking back to that conversation with the nurse, when she asked if there were any questions, why did you respond "no"? Thinking that perhaps even if the answer were yes, would it really make remembering or following these instructions any easier? Let's face it. You don't have a clue about self-managing care.

Reviewing the directions once again and realizing that it is impossible to get in contact with the hospital's nurse, you might feel that the recovery itself is out of reach. And with all the things going on in your house that demand more immediate attention, you find that you are putting yourself last and neglecting to continue the ever-so-important medical guidance that was so carefully delivered. In instances like these, you are not alone. People overlook the importance of self-managing care, especially when it feels like too much, the drive back to the specialist is too long, and the pain and symptoms have subsided for now.

Patient Better makes the ability for proper self-management of care easier. As not too long ago, self-managing care used to be an intangible concept with limited value. It was deemed as non-specific and was too broad of a concept to fit the entire population in need. But today, that is no longer the case, as education for self-managing care has evolved into a patient necessity.

Patient Better brings patients up to speed as to what they can do to better manage their care in this new healthcare-technology era. In fact, it equips you with the necessary skills to help you adjust and improve your health while making a trip to the doctor's office less interruptive of your day.

Now that I am writing this guide within the trenches of the COVID-19 pandemic, I feel compelled to enhance the capabilities of people to self-manage care even more.

I want to supply education to people so that they can manage care for both themselves and for their family members at home and avoid a visit to the healthcare clinic if possible.

I can only achieve this by teaching people with complex conditions and the ones who care for them how to manage and record care for both in-person and [now] virtual medical appointments. I will explain my reasoning throughout this book because as of late, self-managing care has become a requirement for you, your family, and your healthcare team to follow. And together, the three roles of the patient, caregiver, and healthcare professional to have a clear understanding of each other's capabilities while abstaining from face-to-face time as much as possible.

It is so important now to develop a productive relationship and enjoy healthy communication while limiting office visits. This is where most people get confused. Limiting office visits does not mean you are lessening communication with your doctor. Because now, there are many channels of possible communication, people can receive quality medical consultation in the comfort of home. During a crisis or just in everyday life, it is ideal for you to contact your doctor or medical professional through telemedicine services when possible.

Telemedicine is society's answer to many challenges. In this book, you will uncover the amazing concepts and pitfalls of the following:

- Why is telemedicine just emerging into our society and not already a standard in care?
- Why does telemedicine seem limited and not utilized to its full potential?

After reading through the Patient Better Comprehensive Guide to Self-Health Management, you had clarity about many medical terms and the designations of medical practitioners so that no one would ever be able to confuse you. You will never become a victim of misinformation when you are asking the right questions to the right individual. You should feel a lot more confident when communicating about your health. You should now be more self-reliant in your care or providing care to your loved one, and you should be able to independently organize medical care on your own.

Upon reading this book you will be able to transition your newly refined capabilities of self-managing and transition them into a virtual setting. This book helps you understand how to help not only yourself but also your loved one and move from a professionally structured environment into a comfortable controlled setting. You will be a contributing asset in distance, not just a bystander blindly following the directions of your healthcare team. After working with the Patient Better program, you will notice having fewer complications, and it may reduce your number of emergency room visits. You will be prepared for an information-driven appointment every time. As a result, you will be able to minimize unforeseen medical cost.

Contents

Introduction
The Abundance of Health Information

Technology has given us access to information about healthcare like never before. People can more easily retrieve information through the internet, connect with other professionals, and find many ways to improve health and take better care through online or in-person support groups and organizations. As a matter of fact, more and more people are now discovering new solutions to better manage medical conditions just by simply applying proper patient research methods. And as discussed in Patient Better's Comprehensive Guide to Self-Health Management, Article 3.7- Research Smart, most doctors desire their patients to take the initiative to learn how to self-manage care.

As we go through this book, relating to the fact that at no other point in history has there been such an abundance of healthcare information to help patients and caregivers research for care solutions. Access to healthcare instructions has never been easier to obtain, and the "how-to" of caring for oneself has never been so prevalent. It has never been this easy for patients to participate in taking care of their health and overcoming the feeling of not being able to self-manage care on their own. And upon reading this book, you may also find that there are many channels to communicate with healthcare professionals about your condition as well. In turn, and because of heightened communication, caring for your health, aka self-managing care, has never been so sophisticated as it is currently.

Self-managing medical care is a newer concept for most people – maybe even for you. Proper self-management of health is a learning experience. In just the last six years, self-managing care has evolved into a necessary skill for patients to ensure the best possible experience and is the primary driver in furthering one's decision-making competence for health's betterment and quality of life. The Patient Better Self-Health Management Program is to help people from all walks of life with any health condition(s) by offering organizational tools to become better at self-managing care.

Utilizing Health Information to Self-Manage Care

The term "self-managing care" may seem limited because it has the word "self" in it. You might think that healthcare specialists should be responsible for managing your health, and you cannot do justice in treating your condition without complete direction. You must first understand that this presumption will limit your ability to unravel self-managing benefits and really make self-managing work for you.

The term self-managing care is often referred to when an individual creates their own system to manage care for their condition. Healthcare professionals consider self-managing care as a universally applied term used to describe someone who is uncompensated and has no formal training for managing care in any specified condition. These self-taught learners, nevertheless, do their best to manage care for themselves or a loved one and do it completely out of compassion and the benefits that self-governing care bestows.

The idea behind self-managing care remained unclear in the healthcare world until Patient Better. Patient Better standardized a program for the market to have a clear understanding of what a self-managing program does. As not too long-ago self-managing care ranged from one extreme to another (but most people fell somewhere in the middle).

Below are two extreme examples of real-life scenarios of how people would consider themselves to self-manage care:

1. Self-managing care for one person meant that they have meticulously saved every piece of paper and receipt from their treatment. This person chronologically penned down every feeling and ailment they have experienced since they were old enough to start writing.

2. Self-managing care for another meant that they filed their medical paperwork in their car's trunk. After some time, when the ink faded, and the papers weathered the documents were thrown in the trash. This person only found it necessary to keep a memory dialog for as long as they could remember.

In the first scenario, the person gathered excessive information about their health, and for healthcare professionals to collect pertinent data was deemed too time-consuming. In the second scenario, the person's recollection was deemed too unreliable, and without a secure history, it would be impossible for providers to confidently execute an individualized treatment plan. And if I may share a best-kept secret; if the doctor does not have enough information, they will always revert to playing it safe and err to the side of caution.

If you are self-managing care for yourself or your sick loved one without prior experience in the medical industry, undoubtedly, you will find self-managing care challenging. After reading this book you will be able to collect the relevant and pertinent information and organize it in a way to produce a purposeful health story for both in-person and virtual medical appointments. You have identified from the above examples that deciphering and gathering the 'right' information to provide your healthcare provider on your own could turn out to be a time-consuming, confusing, and frustrating task.

The Patient Better program eliminates all such nuisances of learning about the healthcare industry on your own and has developed a program that makes learning about self-managing care unchallenging. You can rely on Patient Better to pave the way for you to organize information about your condition in a manner that, if any future ailments show up, the right documents will be in reach.

Before Patient Better, when a healthcare professional would ask any given patient, "Do you have a self-managing system?" the chances were that the response would be "Yes." For lack of a better phrase that aligned healthcare professionals, insurers, and organizations to understand how their patients collected, organized, and processed paperwork never came to light until Patient Better.

After completing this program, and a provider asks what you are doing to self-manage care your answer to clinicians upgrades to a confident response, "I use Patient Better's system to self-manage care". This means that you are now formally educated to have a more in-depth conversation with your clinician and insurance provider.

You will learn to manage care for yourself or your loved one's medical records in a way that can be effectively used for self-managing. Caregivers will be able to provide better at-home care, and patients will see a massive change in their capability to care for themselves and be able to take on more responsibility while collaborating with experts in their care and living independently longer.

How Self-Managing Care Became a Necessary Skill

We will go further in-depth about this topic throughout the book and connect-the-dots of why self-managing care is now a necessary skill while it may not have been in much demand before. In short, technology replaced medical staff and took over and limited administrative guidance that the healthcare clinic's staff once offered and then transferred the navigation responsibilities onto the unsuspecting patient. Furthermore, the recently in-place electronic software systems have been considered beneficial among the remaining healthcare professionals as it is not as predisposed to errors and oversights as humans.

Documentation management software allowed clinicians to focus specifically on condition management. Electronic recording systems provide healthcare professionals with the opportunity to provide more personalized treatment to their patients by using data retrieval. Through these types of software, professionals can quickly to capture the precise information needed to come up with incredibly accurate solutions. All qualified electronic records documentation systems are secured in HIPAA compliant software and with a good internet connection are easily retrievable by pertinent professionals involved in the patient's care.

Electronic records are also accessible for people that need quick access to their medical records living and working in remote areas far away from their health provider. But at the same time, technology took over and eliminated the need for administrative staff and has moved the operational responsibilities onto the patient's shoulders. So as for today, it is now the patient's responsibility to have online access to retrieve and communicate with providers online.

The Notable Health Concepts of Self-Managing Care

As discussed in Article 1.4 Healthcare Illiteracy- The Hidden Epidemic, medical jargon refers to the terms widely used by healthcare professionals to communicate. Unlike medical terminology, medical jargon is more predisposed to miscommunication as the same word might carry different meanings from one healthcare provider to the next.

When you use medical jargon, it is important for you to distinguish the meaning when speaking to multiple healthcare professionals. The following four essential patient-centric terms have been around for a long time; However, Patient Better has updated these terms' meanings and provided additional value to them. These are terms that all patients and caregivers should be familiar with when self-managing care and should understand their definition to effectively communicate with healthcare providers for fruitful results:

Patient Education

Patient education is a comprehensive term that commonly refers to healthcare professionals providing instruction to patients about a specific diagnosed condition. Patient Better's program is an addition to the traditional education in which you will receive from the clinician. In some cases, you may be the one to introduce Patient Better into the treatment room. So, if a clinician is curious about your Self-Health Manager, please clarify what kind of education you have received from our program. If questioned, our program is referred to as "patient education for self-management."

There are so many benefits to learning how to self-manage care as it is your vessel to heighten your ability to communicate, become more proficient in health literacy, and create a unique story. Indeed, you accomplish this while adopting a more sophisticated medical recording structure in an extremely short amount of time and all while in the comfort of home. Ultimately, the patients who follow the Patient Better program will become more independent and lead a healthier life while improving their health prospects.

Patient Engagement

This term has recently manifested during the time the electronic health records became the new standard for healthcare clinics. Patient engagement typically refers to when the healthcare professional is looking to be more interactive with their patients. Now with self-managing care, it allows for the patient to equally reciprocate interest and to better engage with their professional. So, in patient terms, the word engagement can be defined as the desire and ability to participate in care with your healthcare provider. The provider and patient collectively interact with the same purposeful goal of improving experience and having the most successful end results in care.

What patient engagement means to healthcare professionals is that chronic disease management is a key component in supporting the health care industry's shift toward value-based health care practices. Patient Better utilizes patient engagement in a way that it lets patients follow a specified program, which allows for a more interactive and productive appointment[i].

Self-Managing Care

This term specifies that you are self-managing care for your condition and can be applied for both in-person and virtual medical appointments. In this book, I will emphasize the importance of self-managing care, why it can have an important role in condition management, and how to maintain the quality of care for both in-person and virtual medical office visits.

An Equal Partnership in Care

Your doctor shouldn't be dictating your orders; those days are gone. We briefly touched on the EPIC Relationship in articles 4.1 and 4.2 in The Comprehensive Guide to Self-Health Management. However, in this book, we build on the "patients as partners" concept[ii] as it is an important component to your self-managing care abilities for in-person and virtual medical office visits. And as always, with every healthcare professional that you encounter, you should always remember that the traditional provider-patient relationship should be transformed into the modern EPIC partnership.

With that said, Patient Better has provided additional meaning and value to patients becoming a more intricate part of the care team. With the in-house formula of proper education, increased ability to self-manage care, and being able to proficiently engage with professionals, patients (and caregivers) establish themselves as equal partners. Patients and their caregivers can now work side-by-side with the clinicians to improve their medical condition. The Patient Better program paves the way for patients to play an active role and become an equal partner in the prevention, treatment, and recovery of medical care.

Telemedicine Potential

Today, telemedicine refers to providers and patients interacting through a computer, tablet, or smartphone via Facetime, Hangouts, Skype, or Zoom and other telecommunication lines. Specialties such as neurology, infectious diseases, behavioral health, dermatology, and radiology, are service lines that are commonly covered in telemedicine. Primary care services are also expanding to telemedicine quickly since real-time consultation can involve a quicker diagnosis which telemedicine is well-suited and capable of providing.

Telemedicine offers a simple and often inexpensive solution to diagnosing and treating patients. The healthcare provider communicates with the patient through a screen, and they can connect regardless of the location. Patients save travel costs and reduce their waiting time. This is especially important for patients with conditions that require frequent visits to the clinic and time off work.

Before the pandemic, some employers offer telemedicine services as a benefit while some companies offer remote care right inside the facility. Telemedicine services were scarce, but nevertheless, prided themselves on their offering of intelligent and on-demand access.

The COVID-19 pandemic triggered the need for social distancing and for medical practices to take extra precautionary measures. Medicare and private insurance companies removed the red tape the once limited telemedicine's service capabilities. The hope [with this book] is to provide patients with the knowledge to extend the lifted ban and for third party payers to continue to cover more virtual medical services.

Research shows that telemedicine can be a solution for an underserved population and (if executed properly) has the potential to:

(1) Level inequity and increase access to care.

(2) Improve the efficiency, coordination, and integration of healthcare systems[iii].

Let's unpack these two advantages:

(1) The term inequity of care refers to the underserved population of people that need medical care. These are the folks who live in rural areas and those who have a difficult time leaving the house as opposed to their urban counterparts who live near a medical clinic or hospital and have access to transportation services. Therefore, experts see telemedicine as the answer to providing services to the underprivileged.

(2) Telemedicine can better the healthcare systems in the following ways:

Efficiency: Lowering the expenditures on a brick-and-mortar location such as hiring staff who would provide maintenance to the hospital or clinic. Telemedicine also lightens the health facilities' other costs and expenses as opposed to just having a traditional physical location as it improves patient engagement by extending service hours. People that utilize remote services overall have a positive healthcare experience as they feel providers are more accessible and available for contact at any time, making it easier to establish a closer connection.

Coordination: Traditionally there are limitations of convenience to receive treatment in an 'in-system' network. Meaning that if people stayed within the hospital's network of physicians and ancillary services the patient would have their health information secure and not having to fill out paperwork for each clinician. Today, as telemedicine is coupled with self-managing care, there is more flexibility of choices by expanding the patient's options and accessibility.

Integrating healthcare systems: Self-health management requires data transference through the patient's initiatives. By taking this proactive step, patients and caregivers can expect fruitful outcomes simply by collecting and adequately disseminating their pre-recorded records to each provider.

And through self-managing care, many large hospital systems as well as small independent providers will be able to access uniform patient history to provide effective care. Patients who assist in telemedicine's ability to join health systems understand how patient initiative and record transparency helps with telemedicine's functionality. Furthermore, health information systems' communication is vital for telemedicine services, which undoubtedly improves patient outcomes, and this responsibility also fell upon the patient's shoulders and could potentially become a fundamental characteristic of telemedicine.

A patient who self-manages is also an important component of the health industry's ability to communicate. As the health story tells clinicians and healthcare providers understand the social determinants of their patients' health and how to treat accordingly.

Section One: Building Professional Partnerships

In this chapter, you will learn the fundamentals of patient education of self-management for both in-person and virtual medical office visits. For both patients and caregivers, reading this chapter is the first step to transition your traditional relationship to a modern partnership.

Key Takeaways:

- At the core of self-management are three skills everyone must develop: capable, knowledgeable, and understanding.
- The ability to take control and become a team player and not be afraid to learn new things and advocate for your health care.
- Understand the importance of the EPIC relationship.
- Learn and adapt to new processes.

1.1 Patient Education

Patient education brings meaningful healthcare to patients, enhances the at-home caregiver's capabilities, and supplies a valuable resource to healthcare professionals

Long ago, patient education was considered as the information and instructions that were given by medical staff in a professional environment for the preventative, treatment, or rehabilitative advice about a specific illness, disease, or injury. When patients had questions about their health, they turned to the medical office's staff to understand any health and condition related concerns. In those days, reaching out to a licensed healthcare professional for medical advice was easy to attain.

Patients relied on the medical staff to answer all medical questions that pertained to their bills, make financial arrangements, and discuss in-depth insurance questions. It was common practice for the office's staff members to work together as a team to answer the patient's services, product, or finance queries. And if necessary, the medical staff was allowed to take the extra step to act as the patient's liaison to insurance companies to seek additional guidance as to how the practice and insurer can better assist that patient.

The transition from fee-for-service to value-based practices and the integration of document management systems (DMS) has indeed, helped clinicians deliver higher quality care. As DMS came to the market and promoted its focus on upgrading the office's efficiency and productivity[iv]. DMS has resulted in many practice benefits, and consequently, has also resulted in minimizing staff necessary to perform the same services that were once provided.

Policies and regulations weren't as stringent as they are today. As seemingly just a couple of years ago, clinicians were able to openly discuss on the phone [on a dime and excluded from all the red tape] *medical records*. But today- that is no longer the case.

For various reasons, patient education has extended itself to go well beyond the conversation within the doctor's office. Nowadays, it is common practice for patients to seek answers to their questions outside of the clinic. Whereas earlier, patients were not subjected to a long-automated phone screening just to talk to a live clinician nor did they feel that their question was an interruption. Now, researching is a commonality for both patients and their caregivers to get information from multiple sources outside of the clinic. Health laypeople who conduct their own investigation are becoming aware of the greater need for their healthcare involvement.

Incorporating Family Members in Care and Treatment

Patient education fosters engagement with health providers, financial institutions, and patients[v]. As a reaction to the new value-based clinic patients and professionals realized the impact of incorporating caregivers to take on a more active role and help the patient receive at-home care. Recently health data reviewers observed that the patient's success went hand and hand with the support that they had at home.

The influence of the success was not the number of supporters- but the quality of support that the at-home caregivers provide. The patient reaped the benefits of family member caregivers as at-home observers. In turn, providers became more aware of the patient's environment and underlying circumstance once the patient left their office.

Patient Education Improves Patient and Caregiving Capabilities

These are the components that are incorporated by Patient Better's education to become a successful participant in at-home care. They include communication, literacy, and other key components that are discussed below.

Health Communication– This is the study and practice of communicating in verbal and written form. Communication influences and empowers individuals and families to make healthier selections and make positive changes in attitudes, behaviors, and is the first step to improve health literacy.

Health Literacy- Pertains to the improvement to learn about one's health as well as the surrounding health environment. People who are proficient in health literacy understand the importance of status, use, costs, and outcomes. Health literacy helps patients to understand their own health in a better way and interact with health care professionals on a more engaging level. Patient education and health literacy go hand in hand, and allow laypeople to better understand their condition, medication management, interpret documents, and manage records.

Health Story – This is a meaningful and purposeful detail in a first-person perspective that incorporates all components in one's health, including past and present co-morbidities and therapies. Creating a storyline through the Patient Better system allows you to reduce the chances of having a useful piece of information from being overlooked and triggering further investigations or delay to initiate treatment.

Health History v. Health Story

A patient's health history and health story have a lot in common. Characteristics include similar information such as biographical, demographic, physical, mental/behavioral, sexual, and spiritual data. However, they are not the same. A health history is an overview created by the patient and a licensed practitioner in a professional setting, whereas a health story, is a collection of in-depth (standard and non-standard) details of the health and care throughout a continuum of one's life span and is typically created by the patients and other family members.

Health history pertains to the aspects of the formal care that you have received. A health history may also include a record of information about the individual's prior illnesses, surgeries, and immunizations[vi]. A patient's health history overviews close family members such as parents, grandparents, or siblings that have a current or past illness in their life as well. Detailed information about one's family may include a pattern of circumstances or occurrences that may serve professionals as a predictor for future medical needs.

Whereas a **health story** comprises of more details throughout the journey of one's health. A health story may include the emotional state and underlying behavioral characteristics that are typically excluded from the history's reports and treatments. A health story may also chronicle the patient's lifestyle, as well as the occurrence, and include diet and exercise, socioeconomic changes, death, major life changes and interruptions (divorce), along with personal beliefs.

The Split Patient Education

As we examined earlier, traditional patient education was delivered within the medical practice. However, when clinics evolved from the fee-for-service to value-based practice, so did the way clinicians deliver patient education[vii]. Now, patient education broke up into two parts: (1) education for condition management and (2) education for the administrative duties that co-exist with condition management.

Condition management education

Patient education for condition management is the first part of education that is recognized as the information that one receives in the treatment room. This education remains untouched by the electronic health record and is provided by licensed healthcare professionals (i.e., neurologist, oncologist, rheumatologist, internal medicine physician, or registered nurse)[viii]. Providers of this form of instruction follow a standardized patient-centered education model. The patient-centered instructions are the most widely recognized guidance that provides individualized patient edification. This form of instruction pays close attention to the specific health condition and the individual patient. This type of focus is referred to as patient-centered education and is applied to the patient that was respectful of and responsive to the provider's understanding of the patient's preferences. In the hopes of delivering patient-centered instructions, practitioners would ensure that the patient's values guide all clinical decisions, therefore increasing the chances for the patient to have the best possible outcome.

Administrative education

The second part of education took place after the patient left the treatment room. This education, was (and still is) systematic, meaning that the training is structured and standard. Also, learning the administrative duties is not individualized, unlike patient-centered condition management education. As discussed, a long time back, this education that came after condition management learning was offered by the supporting staff of the clinician and was provided once the patient navigated to the front of the practice. The back-office medical assistant, or liaison, with the patient's chart in hand, would walk the patient to the front of the practice and then hand over the record to another front-desk assistant. The front desk assistant would then further guide the patient in the next steps of care. This secondary form of education was provided by the staff that usually worked in the front of the practice and who would have full access to the patient's complete medical record.

The medical chart allowed staff members to provide direction to the patient as well as the additional guidance of the administrative duties that co-existed with the condition. When the implementation of the electronic health record came in, this part of the patient's education started to vanish. With the electronic health record and the establishment of HIPAA- the paper medical chart disappeared. And today, staff members who work in front of the practice have limited knowledge about the medical status of the patient.

Hence, limiting the front desk's capabilities to supply thorough direction. Indeed, this part of patient education is practically eliminated from practices, but nevertheless, these second instructions serve as a valuable component to better the patient's experience and ability to succeed.

The Distribution of Capabilities and Participation

As discussed in *A Comprehensive Guide to Self-Health Management*, there are two types of participants in the patient's self-management system which are the: (1) individual and (2) contributor. Each participant provides complimenting support qualities. If you recall, the contributor group was then broken down into a hierarchy of roles: clearinghouse, primary caregivers, and secondary caregivers.

Your first assignment is for you and the clearinghouse to get together and establish participation capabilities. The objective of the following diagram is for the individual (patient) and the clearinghouse (the principal contributor) to reflect and work together as a team and recognize each other's participation, contribution needs, or shortcomings. And as always, the clearinghouse represents all contributors and is documented on the Contributor Cover Page. In this activity, the responsibilities of the patient and the clearinghouse are numbered 1-9 in each box.

The goal for the patient and the clearinghouse's numbers (together) should equal ten or greater. If the clearinghouse's and the patient's numbers equal below ten, then the participant's contribution needs to be reevaluated, and each capability of participation should be reanalyzed. This diagram's formula provides a bird's eye view of who needs to enhance their participation, to address the evolving needs of the patient. In other words, this diagram formulizes the patient's and the contributor's capabilities to better complement one another's strengths and weaknesses.

Individual & Contributor Model

#1 Individual (Patient):

Individual (Capabilities)	Group L	Group C	Group T
Mild & Edu. Level 1:	9	6	3
Progressive & Edu. Level 2:	8	5	2
Advanced & Edu. Level 3:	7	4	1

Individual management capabilities # _____

#2 Clearinghouse (Caregiver):

Clearinghouse (Participation)	Group T	Group C	Group L
Mild & Edu. Level 1:	9	6	3
Progressive & Edu. Level 2:	8	5	2
Advanced & Edu. Level 3:	7	4	1

Clearinghouse participation # _____

The patient's capabilities and the clearinghouse's participation combined should equal 10. As shown in the diagrams, the scale ranges from 1 to 9: For both diagrams, nine indicates greater commitment, learning, and organizing demands, and one indicates the least.

_____ The patient's capabilities

+ _____ The Clearinghouse's participation

= _____ Contribution total

Key to Diagram #1

Individual: The individual patient is the person who the self-managing care system is for. This system is centered around the folks who have health issues will address the significance and impactful transitional condition management. Health issues can range on a broad spectrum, from a mild form in development to severe. These conditions may develop late in life or begin before birth. Once Patient Better's Self-Managing Program is acquired, the informal caregiving team will have the knowledge to deliver care properly and consistently, thus, becoming part of a capable care team for both in-person and virtual medical office visits.

Key to Diagram #2

Clearinghouse: Also known as caregivers, family, or friends who are people participating in the self-managing care program and assist patients in their daily activities. Clearinghouses act as the spokesperson for the contributors and continually identify the needs of the patient and are ready to take on more responsibility at any given point of care.

How to Interpret the Row (For both diagrams):

Group L- Lifetime Management

Lifetime management is for those who put self-management into their lifestyle. Group L refers to the folks that are proactive and new to the task of self-managing care. Group L examples would be identified as those who are able to maintain the mild condition that requires long-term management. Lifestyle management may be for ones who need ongoing condition management such as asthma, Crohn's disease, or obesity that introduced you to self-managing care earlier.

Group C- Chronic Condition Management

This group pertains to individuals who have two or more mild to progressive chronic conditions and want to learn the administrative duties for more in-depth self-condition management. These health issues are typically non-aggressive, remain relatively stable, and maybe reversed or go into remission (i.e., diabetes, hypertension, COPD, or cardiovascular issues). However, these conditions may also act as a precursor to more aggressive health conditions like stroke, epilepsy, or heart failure.

Group T- Transitional Condition Management

These are where the mild to the progressive chronic condition has moved into an advanced condition (i.e., Stage two to stage four aggressive cancer, minor aches and pains into rheumatoid arthritis, dementia into Alzheimer's disease) that one can begin in preparation to incorporate contributors if the condition ever requires. These conditions typically demand intensive at-home caregiving management. These patients will then incorporate family members and others to learn how to collaborate effectively with a self-management regimen. Those who suffer from these types of complex health conditions and are enduring these severe illnesses find it extremely difficult to perform daily activities.

How to Interpret the Column

Ultimately, it is up to the licensed professional to diagnose the stage of the health occurrence, the severity of the condition, and the education correspondence necessary for the optimal outcome. This model is a mobile overview for individuals and clearinghouses with the condition that throughout time, the severity will fluctuate. Therefore, the capabilities (expectations) of the patient may worsen or better, and in turn, the responsibilities of the clearinghouse should be reactionary to the patient's health and capability status at any given point in time. However, this status checker also recognizes that if the patient has a mild form of a condition and their capabilities are not affected, then there are no additional requirements in which the clearinghouse needs to provide.

Three Levels of Conditions

Mild: Conditions where one could live without other's help in ADLs, even though the condition exists it does not affect social outings. Examples include diabetes, asthma, high blood pressure, ADHD.

Progressive: May prevent some social gatherings or outings and may seek help with ADLs. Examples include Chronic obstructive pulmonary disease (COPD), a heart condition, arthritis, obesity, glaucoma, dementia, multiple sclerosis.

Advanced: Conditions after which individuals are unable to care for themselves. Examples include severe cognizant disorders, severe brain injuries, late-stage renal disease, and Alzheimer's disease.

Three Levels of Education

There are three levels of administration education in the Patient Better program that is addressed in the Preface but is also a tool to use in this model.

Education Level One- Beginner: The first level is created for those who are new to self-managing. The "Beginner" level focuses on essential education like learning the basics and building a solid foundation of healthcare industry knowledge. The Beginner is designed for people who are healthy and are able to self-manage without assistance. Some diagnosed examples include (pre) diabetes, arthritis, or high blood pressure.

Education Two- Intermediate: This level was created for people diagnosed with complex conditions that may require help from others throughout the occurrence. This level entails "hands-on" training for patients and caregivers for at-home care teams utilized by people with complex condition management demands. Diagnosed examples are heart failure, Alzheimer's disease, cancer, Parkinson's disease, or a major injury.

Education Level Three- Advanced: This level is created for newcomers or advanced levels. The purpose of this level three is to maximize stay at home efforts for in-person and virtual medical office appointments. This level focuses on skills that are needed for telemedicine for complex condition management and at-home team management training for both in-person and virtual medical office visits.

How Patient Education Impacts the Provider-Patient Relationship

One of the basic goals of patient education is to create an environment where patients and caregivers are viewed by healthcare professionals as partners in the care team. Another benefit for patients that work the Patient Better program is to integrate and upgrade the family-member caregivers' capabilities who can assist in the delivery of at-home care. This is the first part of the dynamic of the provider-patient relationship moving into the newer form of the equal exchange of information through the patients enhancing their health communication and literacy skills, creating a health story, and incorporating their family members to help in governing care.

Now that you have taken the next step of acquiring sufficient education about the administrative principles that co-exist with proper condition management you will become more knowledgeable about your care, have more treatment options, and the ability to identify whether it's time to pursue more advanced treatment or therapy.

Education: The First Component to Transform the Provider-Patient Relationship

Patient Better's self-managing program further develops your ability to self-manage care and is your first step to disrupt the traditional provider-patient relationship. As discussed, healthcare communication and literacy affect health status, use, costs, and outcomes. Furthermore, aligning your goals with those of your physician's builds confidence in both parties and puts all involved in care on the same page.

Improves Safety- If you have high-quality communication between the members of your healthcare team, you are able to improve your safety and decrease the risks of oversight. When your physician has a full medical history that includes all your past procedures as well as all your prior conditions, it helps them diagnose and prescribe a safe and effective treatment. Based on previous information and history, your treatment can, therefore, take a lot of the guesswork out of the ability to succeed in treatment.

Improves Experiences- When all members of a team have equivalent education, it diminishes a lot of the guesswork. Education allows patients and caregivers to become a more effective and active part of the care team. Ultimately this education leads to high-quality and improved satisfaction, for everyone, throughout the health journey.

More Efficient Care- Expenses are often a cause of concern for patients when getting a treatment. Patient Better's program ensures to maximize the reduction of expenses for your healthcare. Moreover, improved literacy and communication allows you to have more freedom and continue a professional relationship in a more efficient manner.

Better Outcomes- Self-managing care efforts have led to the patient's ability to become more self-efficient and make more informed decisions and better choices. Thus, improving the patient's outcome. It is recognized that the patient must have a higher sense of self-sufficiency as it plays a major role in how to accomplish goals, tasks, and challenges regarding health.[ix] Clinical benefits in self-managing care have become more prevalent as recent documentation proved within a wide range of conditions such as diabetes, coronary heart disease, heart failure, and rheumatoid arthritis[x].

1.2 An In-depth Self-Managing Program

The Patient Better self-managing system is a meaningful program created to help in communicating your unique health story

As discussed, this administrative education is not just restricted to the conversation inside the treatment room. Healthcare laypeople are having to initiate the second form of training (that no longer exists in the medical practice) on their own. Today, this second part of education is typically self-taught and the knowledge that is learned, one cannot readily share this insight with another. For those [patients and caregivers] who understand this second form of training allows for an enhanced vision of care, but this is only completed on a case-by-case basis. Until Patient Better.

Upon learning the two segments of self-managing care, one's goal is to create an equal relationship, not only between the provider and the patient. If necessary, a self-managing system must also be able to include the caregiver as well. A partnership is cultivated when you take the patient-centered care concept and extend it to the *Relationship-Centered Care* (RCC) model. RCC is an easy transformation as it is applied when an individual patient incorporates at-home caregivers. RCC is the act when the patient and their at-home caregivers acquire the skills and the confidence to govern complex health occurrences

RCC is also part of the EPIC relationship, where it includes the entire health team to participate in care and discuss with professionals on a more meaningful level. This EPIC relationship includes the commitment to assist the patient to attend ongoing assessments, the ability to monitor progress, as well as being able to set achievable goals, and problem-solving- as a team.

Patient Better's self-managing program enables you to not only adhere to the patient-centered model but enhances your abilities. It also allows one to easily incorporate into a team, otherwise known as a relationship-centered model. What this means is that the self-managing program follows suit for you and your caregiving team's education. Not everyone, of course, needs a home care team at this moment. If the need ever arises and you do need help in your daily living activities, this program will help you make incorporating family members more seamless by ensuring that better choices and informed decisions are made throughout care and as a team.

Continuing a united dialog with providers in which all contributors assisting in care responsibilities can obtain an information-driven medical office visit. The more caregivers you have following the Patient Better program, the easier it is for its participants to deliver care and communicate instructions as they update care delivery and the patient's condition changes.

How Learning a Self-Managing Program Became a Necessity for All Associated with Patient Care

Managing a chronic condition is time-consuming and highly complex. Often, it is the patient who is expected to self-manage the broad array of factors that contribute to their health along with the documentation to record and measure outcomes. Research shows that close to 95 percent of individuals with diabetes handle their care themselves entirely. Today, health experts agree that in addition to condition-related education: self-management, continued condition management training, collaborative decision making, goal setting, and problem-solving are also expected from patients to manage care properly. Realistically, the only solution is for patients to enroll in a self-management program that can help individuals and their caregivers boost the care team's ability to manage care.[xi] After all, how could there be a better way to see the patient's unique aspects of health?" Active patient participation provides one with the ability to seek more relevant information about the individual case.

Patient Better's Self-Managing Program Will Bring More Meaning into Your Healthcare

This self-management program empowers you to have more jurisdiction over your choices and decisions regarding your health and well-being. Our relationship-centered care (RCC) model means that team collaboration and coordination make "more at-home eyes that are on the patient- the better." RCC allows the at-home team to help patients keep track of their chronic conditions more closely, stick to their treatment plans, identify, and correct any and all errors as well as contributing quality recordings.

One primary goal of working the Patient Better program is to make your informal caregivers, whom you may have not even known that they could help- assist you in organizing care. Collaborating with an at-home caregiving team is just a fancier way of saying: "Effectively getting your family and friends to help you with your care."

Proficient self-managing skills, for both the patient and at-home caregivers, promote health literacy and communication, increases compliance which results in more cost-effective and efficient healthcare delivery, and reduces complications related to the illness.[xii] No matter how great or how small the task is, with the betterment of self-managing skills the patient and caregiver can ensure a better health experience.

Case Scenarios

1. A granddaughter that can drive

Let's say that you are unable to drive to the doctor's office on your own, and your children are working. However, your granddaughter, who knows how to drive, gets out of school in enough time but is unsure of what information or paperwork is relevant to the appointment. Normally, your children would have to take off work to ensure that the appointment is productive.

Patient Better's solution would be to prepare your granddaughter for the appointment with you the night before the visit and have your Self-Health Manager ready. On the day of the appointment, your children wouldn't have to leave work, and you can attend the appointment with your Self-Health Manager alongside your granddaughter.

During your medical visit, make sure that you direct your healthcare professionals to submit relevant information into the communication pocket of your Self-Health Manager so that your children can take a look at it when they get home.

2. Caring for a child

Your child has a speech impediment, and they need therapy to overcome it. You are a single parent, so taking off work and going to a physical location three times a week to visit a speech-language pathologist is not a realistic option.

Patient Better would save you from this life complexity by guiding you in the steps needed to execute long-term therapy. How to alert your daycare employees or babysitter of all the requirements to conduct therapy online and what is required of them. A self-management program gives you the ability to make provisions if necessary, such as bringing an iPad with earbuds along to the sitters and letting them know the importance for your child to have a quiet place to learn. Thus, making it possible to get your child's therapy without physically visiting the therapist.

3. Caring long-distance

Your mother was recently diagnosed with dementia, and you live and work three hours away. However, due to your hectic schedule, you can only visit your mother for two weekends a month. Your goal is to keep your mother living in her house for as long as possible. Your doctor has given you their recommendations and instructions, and you are very aware that the progression of this disease is unpredictable. You also realize that it is essential to hire home care services that can assist your mother in daily activities.

In this case, a home care team will help you fulfill your goals for your mother is to supply your Patient Better program to everyone who visits and contributes care. Show the home care representatives the necessary documentation and communication required of the program and have them agree to follow directions. Make sure that you let as many people as possible know about your self-management program so that your mom is not devoid of care while battling dementia and you are not left in the dark.

4. Caring for sick parents as a child

Taking adequate care for sick parents is not an easy task. Statistics show that kids who care for ill parents are less likely to perform well in school, have a more difficult time caring for themselves, and face difficulties when they undergo the transition into adulthood.

This is an extremely tough topic unless you are a doctor, social worker, counselor, or insurer who helps in this line. Patient Better offers our program and extends training to all healthcare providers involved in the ailing parent and the child who cares for them as well as the entire home care team.

Self-Health Management the Second Component to Modernize the Provider-Patient Relationship

By the end of this article, you will know how health literacy, communication, and creating a health story helps with your ability to self-manage care. This overview is the foundation that you want to establish when governing all office visits along with the first component (patient-education and taking the patient-centered care model and extending the RCC model) to form an EPIC relationship. The self-management education along with the extension of care is designed for those specifically with ongoing health conditions and get family and friends to better participate in healthcare, and organize documents and take that additional help for all involved in at-home care to live their life to the fullest.

Care Coordination and Contribution from Participants

Care coordination equips patients to develop the care team at home who can participate in making informed decisions — serving as an extension of the primary providers' office-based care team members who are interacting and monitoring patients in between office visits and providing at-home information of progress and status.

An at-home care coordination system cultivates frequent and extremely accurate information about patient's treatment history, medication adherence, new symptoms, and maintenance of chronic conditions in addition to insights to mental health and well-being as well as social determinants of health. With more at-home data supplied with care coordination, providers typically see clinical outcomes improve for the patients that they serve.

Self-Health Managing as an At-Home Team and Utilizing Technology

The ability to self-manage care gives you the tools that are essential to organize standard and non-standard medical care for both in-person and [now] virtual medical office visits. And today, Patient Better is there for you to keep up with the current trends. Just a few years ago, the healthcare industry was struggling to organize telemedicine and bring it to the market.

Today, it is not only convenient but also a necessity for the people who are residing in urban areas as well as for those who live in rural areas.

As far as digital literacy is concerned, it is closely attached to health literacy. It points toward the ability of the patient or their caregivers to maintain their own health as well as the healthcare system. Digital health literacy impacts the patient's ability to use the patient portal or electronic health record.

1.3   Intro to Digital Health

Introduction to health technology, digital records, and managing at-home administration duties that co-exist with today's expanded healthcare service delivery methods

How the Digital Healthcare Clinic Came to Be

To reduce healthcare costs and make healthcare more affordable, our healthcare system identified efficient, cost-effective, and sustainable ways to lower US health spending. Among the many sources of high spending within the United States, is the administrative costs that support the direct costs for services. To make healthcare more affordable, our industry tamed the direct costs and provided additional protection to the patient by implementing health information technology (HIT). Efficacy for implementing HIT into the medical practice has proven successful, but the drawback to this was that medical clinic's administrators were replaced with kiosks, electronic health records, bill processing companies, and other technologies.

The focus to implement HIT into the medical practice was to reduce the costs while not affecting the clinician's ability to deliver quality care. Although reducing the administrative staff has not affected direct patient care the downside of this implementation of technology transfer of the administrative duties from the office staff, which inevitably fell onto the shoulders of the patient.

How Technology Improves Patient Care, Efficiency, Effectiveness, and Safety

Value-based practices, otherwise known as pay-for-performance practices, utilize many forms of technology as well as DMSs as a solution to increase the quality of care, patient safety, and document more thorough outcomes. DMS is a parent term for electronic health record (EHR) or electronic medical record (EMR) systems. When DMSs are implemented into the clinic, this form of technology becomes the infrastructure of the medical practice.

The functionality of DMS is not just limited to documenting medical records electronically, as its name implies. It also plays a significant role in helping physicians improve communications and interactions with their patients[xiii]. This medical technology not only allows the physician to enhance their patient's experience of the encounter but also enables the practitioners to see the whole medical picture, thereby bridging any gaps across the patient's entire health history.

Electronic Medical Records Explained

The practice's online portal is part of the office's electronic recording software. This technology is the provider's way to help you get into their practice without having to physically step into their clinic. Ultimately, it's the patient's responsibility to take action for enrolling themselves in each medical office's portal. So if you haven't done so already, setting up your online portal(s) is the first step to self-manage care for both in-person and virtual medical office visits. It is a necessary job and can be completed with a little diligence.

Two Ways to Enter the Physician's Office

Think of each medical office's portal as the online door to the practice. Each medical office's physical door is different from the next. And so is each clinic's portal. Each door and medical practice have specificities that making entering and exiting unique, however; all doors, like medical practices, serve the same purpose.

Now let's imagine a physician's office's entrance and what their door would look like to their online portal. Most likely if your doctor is operating a value-based practice, chances are they offer an elaborate DMS where registration and scheduling are encouraged and is the preferred path of communication. And you can envision their door being largely made of the finest oak and iron-clad handles.

Whereas another physician may offer a simple online portal as their door would have a modest look created for function and purpose. You imagine a door that is already inside a building, with a sign that reads "No Soliciting," which is suited for the office and the high volume of solicitors rushing back and forth right outside. Indeed, just like the physical door to the medical practice, the portal is the passage to the record management system. Each corridor provides you with the ability to easily enter and exit the office accordingly.

The physician's online portal is not only the entryway to the DMS it is also an extension of service's offering intended to add value to their practice. The online gateway enables you to better engage with your physician as well as help you manage your condition without physically being there. The healthcare facility's portal is a key component in self-managing and virtual medicine.

Limitations of Technology

Technology is a blessing for humankind, but it has limitations as well. However, the DMS is tethered to each practice unable to transfer from one system to the next. While that may be efficient for the individual practice, it is not realistic for patients with multiple conditions to have one professional to provide all care to one individual. Proper care management in one's life span requires multiple clinicians and specialists to deliver individualized services that will cover diagnosis that may arise.

Realistically, you will go to multiple physicians throughout your life, you will move, practitioners will retire leaving you to seek care that meets your individualized needs at any given time. The more conditions that you manage, the more professionals are involved in your care. And without proper self-management, the more at-risk you become to losing unified health information and a greater chance for that information to become diluted. A perfect example of the limitation of the technology is that you may remember telling one healthcare professional one thing, but it may have been the wrong person to tell that (maybe important) information to. And because of various privacy concerns, the healthcare provider may or may not, bring that to your attention.

Whether you decide to self-manage care, or not, the burden of health information transference's weight rests completely on your shoulders. As today most clinicians leave it up to their patients to tell the appropriate person. This is yet another factor of complexities and adhering regulations and ever-advancing technology limitations. Everyone has to compromise and make sacrifices due to these limitations.

The Healthcare Clinic and the Adaptation of Documentation Management Systems

Going back to the door analogy being a gateway to the office, the physician's portal is the online entrance to their DMS. Like the purchase of a door, there are several DMSs that your provider can choose from. Each physician will determine their electronic record need and examine each record's system's particular features and offerings. Some doctors look for function and charm while others look for beauty and ostentation. The system that your physician chooses will most likely reflect their practice's services offering and the facility owner's personality.

As calculated a purchase that a documentation management system will be for the clinic, in the long run, it is the office's goal to have a system's benefits to override the cost. Today, the office's DMS's information stays within the clinic. However, it is the goal that one day that each doctor's office's technology will have a way to communicate with one another. Clinics are preparing for this transaction of patient data by simulating their organization's workflow, participating in the physician quality reporting system (PQRS), and ensuring that their patients get the right care at the right time.

The Future Benefits of Technology

Let's take the example that you have a condition of knee osteoarthritis. After years of your primary physician keeping an eye out on the progression, they have determined that additional attention was necessary. They have referred you to a specialist. The specialist provided consultation and needed additional diagnostic services and determined a diagnosis that required knee replacement surgery.

In order for the surgeon to provide your insurer with documented medical necessity, they needed the current lab report and image. The surgeon also wants you to have the best possible experience so they will provide a place to perform the surgery with an overnight stay at the hospital for further monitoring. At the end of the day and aside from your primary provider's patient portal, you have acquired six more portals, including the specialist's, the diagnostic facility, the lab, the hospital/surgery center, home healthcare, and rehabilitation therapy.

Yikes! That's a lot of portals, but it's important for you to log in to each one of them because ultimately, those records are stored and may need your attention. This may not look like an advantage now, but the patient portals have a host of benefits. Ultimately, it is the goal of the industry to have a seamless transaction of patient data disseminated from clinic to clinic. Currently, the patient's willingness to interact with the office's portals is what we have right now. So, even though multiple portals might be difficult to manage, it is in your best interest to leverage the online offering for your benefit.[xiv]

DMS's Features and Benefits for Patients:

Features

- You can view your test results.
- You can request prescription refills.
- You can pay your bills.
- Instant message- a glimpse of whether the doctor will want you to come in or if the appointment can be conducted remotely.
- You can schedule an appointment and get reminders via email/text as well as updates on the appointment status, cancelation, or rescheduling lock-ins.
- You can retrieve medical documents for further care and keep documentation for insurance purposes.

Benefits

- Your healthcare provider has a better chance to provide accurate, up-to-date, and complete information.
- You will have quick long-distance access to your record.
- You will have additional security for your health.
- More reliable and safer prescriptions.

- Healthcare convenience, improved efficiency, and encounter productivity.
- Legible streamlined notes, improved safety, reduced duplication of testing and decreased paperwork.

The Impact of DMS and the Provider-Patient Relationship

The traditional provider-patient relationship resembled a parent-child association. However, it has now been reconstructed to a more reciprocating interaction; it is more of a mutual partnership. Patient Better's self-managing program allows us to evolve the provider-patient relationship conscientiously and effectively into a modern exchange of information. Digital health has also paved the way for supporting the modern relationship as well.

This shift, proven through multiple studies, suggests that patients now prefer to coordinate care via a more corresponding exchange of treatment decisions with their provider. As the readiness of healthcare information progresses, an extension of telemedicine services evolves, and the delivery of medical services continues to advance, patients prefer an equal partnership. As this equal partnership is becoming more prevalent, it is crucial that patients as well as their families position themselves as active participants in care as a team and must ensure that they remain cognizant of their medical record and health at all times.

Patients have expressed a need to incorporate their family member caregivers in their healthcare processes.

As healthcare advances, these family member caregivers are expected to perform more sophisticated at-home care. Consequently, a transformation took place in the desire for caregivers to have a more corresponding synergy with their loved one's provider as well.

This happened when [along with additional responsibilities of care delivery] two primary contributors of technology occurred: (1) the implementation of electronic health records within the practice. (2) the patient's access to health information (via social media, google, and other technological platforms). Today, in the era of information overload, people are more exposed than ever to all kinds of health information via various channels. This, combined with the expectation to self-manage care, provokes us to question: *"Why wouldn't there be a shift of the provider-patient relationship?"*

Sure, patient education for self-managing care is different from the education that you receive in the treatment room, but it is just as necessary in order for you to have the best possible outcome. In comparison, licensed professionals provide you with individualized education that is specifically about your condition and how to manage it. Patient Better supplies you with the administrative knowledge of your care.

Keeping in mind that the overall medical costs may vary from one health occurrence to the next, the administration's responsibilities will not change; it will just transform the patient into an informed advocate for one's health and the most valuable player on the healthcare team. Therefore, refining the provider-patient relationship into what it is today.

What happened

Before the implementation of the practice's electronic health recording system, the patient-centered education delivery methods were relevant and could be executed seamlessly within the medical practice. When technology entered the healthcare sector, the consequence of this implementation eliminated the administrative positions within the practice. Today, those jobs are non-existent, and apart from paying a co-pay or deductible, patients who have complex health conditions most likely have a sophisticated financial model that is predisposed to oversight or error. Today, people are expected to learn the administrative duties that co-exist with their condition and be responsible to do it on their own.

Section Two:
Telemedicine Services

This chapter was created for you and your at-home caregivers to get familiar with telemedicine's delivery services. In this chapter, we find out how to maintain continuity of care through telemedicine services, know exactly what to do to avoid delayed care, and safeguard ourselves from the consequence of postponing care.

Key Takeaways:

- Knowing what services telemedicine currently offers and how its operations enable people who need additional medical consultations, get them.
- Understand how to access providers, specialists, and behavioral health service providers to better manage chronic conditions.
- Access more support care and address unique underlying factors to receive management of individualized conditions
- Fully take part in physical therapy, occupational therapy, and other modalities as a hybrid approach to optimize convenience, health, and care
- Better post-surgical and encounter follow-up capabilities (especially for the long-distance patient and those with limited mobility)

2.1 The Patient's Guide to Proper Telemedicine

An overview of telemedicine services, their uses, benefits, and how they are relevant to self-managing care

For the most part, telehealth and telemedicine have interchangeable meanings. These two terms can be universally applied, as they both refer to the distribution of health-related services via telecommunication technology. Through this intel, telemedicine and telehealth can mean anyone involved can contact, advise, educate, and monitor via remote admissions of medical care.[xv]

Telehealth and telemedicine are medical jargon and used in many scenarios for healthcare laypersons. You will find that many written reports directed to patients communicate telehealth and telemedicine to mean the same. However, the professionals use the word telehealth to articulate when a healthcare professional completes e-learning, updates, or exchanges information remotely to and from other professionals. Whereas telemedicine is typically applied when describing the interaction and exchange of information between the patient and the professional. Telemedicine specifically refers to the meaning of virtual communication so that the long-distance patient, their chosen healthcare professional, or other clinicians can exchange information.

So, for clarity, we will use telehealth when describing the interaction between healthcare professionals like in store-and-forward/asynchronous communication services. And we will refer to telemedicine when referring to the exchange of information between the patient and the professional like real-time or synchronous communication.

There are two forms of telecommunicating in medicine (A) Asynchronous telecommunication where communication is delivered and examined later and (B) Synchronous telecommunication, whereas the provider and patient exchange information in a live setting. You can remember the difference between asynchronous and synchronous by envisioning that you have to sync together in real-time, and async is not necessary to have asynchronous communication. There are three primary types of remote healthcare services: (1) store-and-forward services, (2) interactive/real-time communication, and (3) remote patient monitoring.

A. Asynchronous telecommunication

Store-and-forward services

From a patient's perspective, store-and-forward services, otherwise known as asynchronous communication, refers to provider-to-provider communication. Real-time communication between the receiver and the sender is not required in this form of communication. Store-and-forward services refer to the act when healthcare providers share information for the other to review later.[xvi]

Asynchronous communication usually happens between medical professionals to assist them in the diagnosis and further examination, especially when they don't require live video or face-to-face contact. Store-and-forward services allow the electronic transmission of medical information such as diagnostic images, digital photos, video clips, documents, and other patient data through secure email. Physician-to-physician or professional-to-physician communication is normally performed to use already collected information, evaluate cases, or render services outside of real-time interaction. Store-and-forward services are mostly used in radiology, dermatology, and ophthalmology.

The benefit of store-and-forward technologies for patients and providers is that they can get additional insight into the diagnosis without traveling beyond the location of the healthcare professional. Wait times for results are decreased. Regardless of their location, providers and specialists can review patient cases and do not have to synchronize work time schedules with others. This leaves professionals with an ample amount of time for research and data collection outside business hours.

B. Synchronous telecommunication:

Interactive/Real-time communication

Interactive or real-time communication is also called synchronous communication and refers to the communication between the clinician and the patient. Synchronous care is ever-evolving, and HIPAA compliance concerns are at the forefront of the professional's mind. And, in light of privacy concerns, only designated interactive audio and visual equipment is utilized in real-time communication for video conferencing between the clinician and patient. But with most insurances adhering to the pandemic's lifted ban, you can complete a real-time telemedicine appointment with applications like Zoom, Skype, Hangouts, or FaceTime. The two forms of real-time communication scenarios are 1) where the patient completes a virtual appointment in their home or 2) the patient completes the office visit from an already medically established setting. These designated places are known as *hub and spoke* and have access to the main campus.

Asynchronous and Synchronous Communication:

Remote patient monitoring

From the patient's perspective, telemonitoring implies using technology in place of self-testimony. Common remote monitoring happens when the patient is discharged from the hospital and goes home but the doctor still needs to continue monitoring health. Remote patient monitoring allows the provider to carefully monitor their patients while they continue to recover in the comfort of home. Today there are many devices where physicians can gather and share vital information and make necessary adjustments if needed.

Monitoring of this type is often used to manage patients at high risks, like those with heart conditions. Not just heart conditions, but remote monitoring has been found to be highly useful for the treatment of several chronic conditions. Diabetic patients can utilize it to track their glucose levels and elderly patients at home or in assisted living facilities who need monitoring. Some examples of remote medical devices include an electrocardiogram (EKG), ultrasound, dermatoscope, and a pulse oximeter.

An Overview of Telemedicine Service Providers

Throughout your journey in self-managing care, you will encounter different telemedicine service providers similar to in-person care. Much like the numerous support staff we discussed within the brick and mortar practice in Patient Better: The Comprehensive Guide to Self-Health Management, the clinicians that you speak via telecommunicating will also have a technology-based staff working behind the scenes. And like the staff in a physical location, the virtual staff, sorted into two groups, ensure that you have the most pleasant encounter and experience possible.

(Group One) Standard Providers

Are the state's licensed healthcare professionals to deliver and oversee medical care and services for the prevention, diagnosing, treatment, and recovery of health predicaments.

Primary care providers include professionals like family practitioners, internal medicine physicians, or licensed pediatricians, and the state-recognized professionals to serve you as the primary overseer of your health. They have an established relationship with you and have full access to your medical record and health history.

Specialty physicians are physicians that dedicate themselves to a particular line of medical examination. Specialists provide more attention to a pertinent diagnosis within a particular line of study and work inconjunct with primary providers.

Like primary care providers, specialists write medical notes (that can be held up in a court of law), prescribe medication, diagnose, and provide treatment. Examples would be (1) a neurologist to treat Parkinson's disease, (2) a rheumatologist to treat arthritis, or (3) a gastroenterologist to treat acid reflux disease, or (4) a urologist to treat incontinence. To receive telemedicine services, specialists also require a face-to-face meeting before tele-treatment and may also require a referral to treatment.

Ancillary Care Service Providers- They are the supporting staff that is trained in diagnostic imaging, therapy, drawing blood, or read reports to aid professionals to further diagnose or treat patients.

Online urgent care or doctor-on-demand- These are the doctors who will only provide short-term treatment online and do not perform follow up appointments. Because of just being restricted to online technology, they are limited in treatment options and can only supply limited condition management.

(Group Two) Non-Standard Providers

Are informal caregivers and company representatives that assist the patient with at-home daily living activities. They are individuals who are not licensed by the state to diagnose illness, injury, or disease.

At-home Caregivers (Informal Caregivers) are unpaid volunteers that are not formally trained and do not receive income to help you in your daily living activities. They are often considered to be your family, friends, or neighbors, or anyone else in your social group that helps you in some way with your daily living activities.

Home Care Caregivers are the paid and trained employees who do not render medical services but instead assist people in executing their daily living activities. Home care agency representatives' assist the patient with essential daily activities and maintains the quality of life by helping to walk, bathe, dress, and provide companionship.

Telemedicine Patient Services Uses

As far as usage and adaptability are concerned, telemedicine is still in its infancy stage. However, telemedicine has recently shown enormous potential to become a fast, reliable, and effective standard of care. It can help people have more access to healthcare, enhance health outcomes, and reduce chronic condition management costs.[xvii] Studies that have been conducted that compared telemedicine technology to traditional medicine and highlight that telemedicine has an economic benefit, especially for those who live in rural areas and strive to live independently longer. At the same time, it reduces emergency room visits, hospital admissions, re-admissions, and the length of stay.

Chronic disease management

Around 57 million Americans live in rural areas, and of that, twenty percent of all healthcare spending comes from those who reside in rural areas. Whereas seventy-five percent of healthcare spending is dedicated to treating heart disease, diabetes, and cancer and that lion share of the people who are at-risk for these conditions are elderly. As a result, telemedicine technology enables physicians to monitor the conditions more closely. In addition to self-health management, their caregivers and other care professionals can collaborate with the patient's care schedule and families.

(A) Monitoring patient changes

Those diagnosed with long-term illnesses often make changes to their lifestyle to improve their health situation. By increasing patient's access to specialized care and reducing travel expenses, they can now seek care regularly and get the well-deserved care and attention they need.

(B) Triage new symptoms in real-time

For patients with chronic conditions, it's not uncommon for them to experience new symptoms over time. These symptoms could either indicate a minor concern or a signal that the patient's health is further deteriorating.

Ultimately, when patients are not within their familiar physician's reach, chances are they will postpone diagnosing and apt not to consult with their physician until the issue is exacerbated. Nevertheless, they took a risk to wait and see. This circumstance happens all too often when traveling long distances, and there is no other option left but to seek immediate care from an unfamiliar source and usually extremely costly price. However, if the already established provider-patient relationship is communicated through telemedicine- then perhaps the patient would have been able to rectify concerns as they become worse.

Medication management

Medication management is an extremely important topic, especially when we talk about seniors. People who are older are at more risk to forget about their prescribed medications. Healthcare professionals can now use telemedicine to help at-home caregivers monitor whether patients have taken their medicines and offer electronic reminders. This kind of collaboration ultimately leads to fewer complications, re-admissions, and improves compliance.

Medical information sharing

Store-and-forward services have been a big game-changer in enabling healthcare providers to connect with other specialists over long distances. All the diagnostic images, lab results, and more can be shared and consulted via asynchronous communication.

Emergency room diversion

The emergency room has the most stressful environment among any other health setting and is the most expensive and overcrowded department. For patients, the financial repercussions can be tremendous, as research shows that a significant portion of those visits can also be avoided. Studies show that 30% of all emergency care (and costs associated with this care) is non-urgent. If telemedicine is utilized properly, it usually only takes three to four minutes of conversation to receive quality guidance to self-manage care. Usually, an urgent care professional can tell within the first 30 seconds whether you need to go to a facility in-person. If you are uncertain whether your ailment requires a trip to the ER, then an urgent care call is your best bet to determine if an in-person exam is avoidable.

Costs for emergency care can increase quickly, and afterward, your insurance company may claim that your ER visit was not an actual emergency. When that happens, people are left to pay high-deductibles or co-pay emergency treatment for a non-emergency issue.

NICU/ICU

A significant decrease in additional in-office visits and calls from worried patients was observed by healthcare facilities that offer telemedicine follow-up visits. These take place after the baby is discharged. This form of telemedicine can be used in a variety of ways. There is no more need to transfer high-risk infants to other locations as they can be seen by specialists from other facilities.

Disaster relief

When any disaster occurs, emergent and non-emergent care is provided by the local healthcare resources that are pulled in. For instance, during Hurricane Harvey and the COVID-19 pandemic, healthcare professionals were able to provide virtual non-emergency care and behavioral health consultations; and it jump-started telemedicine's value into high gear. Thus, shifting medicine's priorities and enabling practitioners to focus on in-person emergency demands. During states of an emergency such as these examples, it is extremely resourceful to determine what occurrence is urgent and care which can be managed remotely.

Paramedic/Ambulatory

Once an emergency department reaches its capacity, it is usual for it to shut down its doors. As a result, ambulances have to transfer patients to other hospitals that are located far away. By using telecommunication, paramedics can find out the capacity of the emergency room in real-time. They don't need to take the patient to a hospital only to have them transferred again to another facility.

Telemedicine for remote clinics

Like hub and spoke clinics or retail clinics like Walmart or Target, the pharmacy department has kiosks available where you can have a real-time office visit for a consultation with an on-demand physician. After you type in your symptoms through a touchscreen computer, you enter a virtual waiting room and get connected with a physician in no time.

Mobile health

Smartphones have played a pivotal role in remote monitoring. Today, small scopes and other peripherals can easily plug in and turn the mobile phone into a diagnostic tool and point-of-care tests that can be easily carried around.

Modern health consumers utilize their smartphones and are accustomed to downloading apps for virtual office visits. With telecommunication technology, e-visits can be accomplished with just a few clicks, and a patient can choose a physician with whom they could speak, message, and video conference.

The Benefits of Virtual Medicine Services

Save the costs and time of transportation

When you have a virtual visit with your physician, you save money on wear and tear on your vehicle, tolls, gas, and parking. Even better, you save your traveling time and save yourself from getting stuck in a traffic jam, which makes you late for your medical appointment or getting back to work.

No need to take time off from work

When we talk about your professional career, telemedicine relieves a big chunk of time that you would need otherwise to make that appointment. You can make a virtual medical office visit during your break. You can even take a little time from your lunch hour. With telemedicine, most physicians will offer extended hours, so you can simply schedule an office visit before or after work so long as you are somewhere that offers sufficient privacy. If you follow Patient Better's self-health management program, you can effortlessly deal with your doctor's follow-up instructions and maintain your health without missing a day of work or spending any additional time.

Eliminate childcare or eldercare issues

Ensuring adequate health care for yourself and for your family members, especially children and elders is vital. However, when you are in need or the ones that you care for are in need of an exam and the only option to physically visit a medical office; it is difficult. Taking other people's needs into considerations while upholding your own commitments is not always an easy task. A meeting with the physician remotely when possible solves many challenges.

Greater access to more specialists

When diagnosed with a serious health condition, the sensible option is to choose the best doctor rather than the doctor who is nearby. Virtual medicine and self-health management make leveraging the expertise of specialists accessible (those you normally would not have access to) for you and your primary provider.

Less chance of catching a new illness

While we all do our best to prevent catching an illness, a crowded waiting room increases the likelihood of a disease being transferred from one individual to another. By leveraging virtual medicine services, you will easily receive the care you need, all the while, avoid unnecessary exposure, thus mitigating your chances of getting yourself and someone else infected with a contagious illness.

Decreased waiting room time

Hospitals and health clinics strive to make their facilities more accessible, personable, and efficient. If you choose a telemedicine visit, you'll be eliminating the largest source of stress from the equation of the in-person office visit.

Get a second opinion

It doesn't matter what type of health issue you are facing. It could be a complex issue or the treatment decision could be extremely difficult. You can easily get a second opinion and ensure that you make well-informed decisions about your health and wellbeing.

Have Better Health

There are many benefits to proper self-management and visiting a care specialist. First of all, you can get rid of any and all physical challenges like getting to the office. Secondly, you can maintain your lifestyle better without any hindrances[xviii].

TELEMEDICINE SERVICES

2.2 Current Challenges in Telemedicine

Taking a closer look at the challenges of implementing, training, and adopting telemedicine into the healthcare marketplace

As we discussed, there are many advantages in telemedicine's offering along with a wide range of potential benefits. Yet, from a clinician's standpoint, there are some risks and challenges regarding service delivery via remote medicine as well. Private and public practice's implementation concerns, for various reasons, differ from one another, however; the end result of the clinic's patient's adaptability will remain the determining factor for the practice's success in implementation[xix].

While physicians are expected to uphold telemedicine's already set standards to deliver remote care that is equivalent to in-person treatment. There are many contributions that the patient must commit to having a continuum of telemedicine appointments.

This is a tricky situation to discuss because I have run into people that just simply refuse to learn how to work on the computer. Granted, the same individuals will easily and gladly Facebook and video chat with family, but anything perceived as outside of the immediate benefits- those users are reluctant to use. Please don't be one of those people, but if you are, ask a friend or family member to help you get started with telemedicine and self-managing. From what I can ascertain, and in my research writing this book, telemedicine has made itself just as easy to work as social media.

Below is a checklist of essential understandings that would help to implement telemedicine into your home easier:

- ✓ Understand the state-to-state licensing limitations.
- ✓ General idea to determine which situations are more appropriate for in-person visits.
- ✓ Comfort level in disclosing personal information outside the closed doors of the treatment room.
- ✓ Access to appropriate technology or connectivity.
- ✓ Comfort level of handling technology (or having someone to help).

Below are the concerns that every potential telemedicine provider has on their mind:

1. Fear a breakdown of the continuous connections and long-term relationships with their patients.

2. Skepticism over potential incomplete health history or the lack of access to the patient's complete medical record.

3. Additional communication complexities, confusions, and not being fully able to retain their patient's individualized needs.

By having the above checklist completed, you will ensure an ongoing cohesive relationship with your clinician[xx].

Relationship Models

Familiarize yourself with the following relationship models. It becomes necessary to understand the active-passive model at times. The guidance-cooperation model and the mutual-participation model are the two primary interactions between patients and physicians in communicating for both in-person and virtual medical office consultations. As for self-managing care for both in-person and virtual medical office visits, it is imperative to incorporate mutual participation in care when building a health provider relationship.

Self-managing care is the first step to evolve the traditional provider-patient relationship or into an EPIC Partnership. Being able to self-manage care, coupled with promoting and responding positively to an EPIC partnership, is the recipe providers and patients need to make the in-person and virtual medical appointments work.

Three dimensions of provider-patient interactions

The Active-Passive Model

The active-passive model is based on the patient being solely acted upon by the physician. This relationship is appropriate when the patient is unconscious or incapacitated and unable to make decisions for themselves. It applies when irreversible and unrecoverable harm might come from a delay in treatment.

Guidance-Cooperation Model

The guidance-cooperation model is a relationship structure when the physician takes on the parent's role, and the patient takes on the role of the child. The physician decides the most appropriate treatment recommendations based on what they believe is in the patient's best interest. In return, it is expected that the recommendations will be complied with by the patient.

Mutual Participation Model

This relationship relies upon the mutual exchange of treatment decisions between the patient and the physician. The patient is thought of as an expert in their life's experiences and goals, and it is the physician's role to help the patient attain these goals. As there is a mutually interdependent exchange of activities, this model needs a higher patient involvement level[xxi].

Relationships and Partnerships Explained

As technology undergoes more advancements, healthcare professionals are continuing to rely on you and your ability to communicate and transfer relevant information from one clinic to the next. A self-management program connects the dots of responsibility and uncertainty to make the mutual participation model work. The Self-Health Manager is your transparent health story and furthers the accessibility of uniformed health information to all members of your care team. When building trust in the participation model it is important to have a prepared health story when you have a consultation with your PCP and that they are aware of your self-management intentions.

Exploit your self-management to its full potential and utilize your primary care physician to help guide you to convey health data to your specialist. Utilizing your PCP in this manner supplies you with an enormous advantage in getting the right diagnosis in the shortest amount of time. Physicians are getting short on time due to the excess workload and higher-volume caseload. The more concise information you provide clinicians from the very start, the more a professional can execute a decisive treatment plan.

The traditional Guidance-Cooperation Model

Patient Better's: Guild to Self-Health Management emphasized the significance of being prepared for the in-person medical appointment. At the same time, it provided a solid foundation for the guidance-cooperation model for functional in-person treatment. But this model has its limitations. In this model, the doctor is in a position of power. They have all the medical knowledge and the patients are completely dependent on the doctor, who can decide what is beneficial for the patient. The patient is then is expected to fully comply with the recommendations and instructions. This model does not work for a virtual appointment because (I will explain further in part three) it takes a higher level of commitment on the patient's part to organize records, complete the pre-assessment before the appointment, along with keeping a good document trail after the encounter and become partners with their third-party payer.

The Modern Mutual Participation Model

In virtual medicine, the mutual participation model works best. In this model, the patient is not just a passive recipient of recommendations and orders but is considered to be an expert in his or her life experiences and goals[xxii]. This makes patient involvement absolutely vital. The physician is not the authority but a helper and a guide whose aim is to help the patient achieve his or her goals. It is especially so if you want to make the most out of telemedicine and meet advanced treatment goals. This also applies if you wish to remain independent for as long as possible or to complete as much of the recovery on your own and continue assistance from insurers[xxiii].

Let's consider these three scenarios:

1.Leslie Smith's Case:

A 37-year-old single female with one 13-year-old child, she works as a full-time accountant. Ms. Smith consults one primary care physician who oversees her full medical record and her condition of type 2 diabetes. She also has two specialists for GI track concerns and a urologist for incontinence.

Just by self-managing care, Leslie prepares for each virtual medical appointment, and she communicates with all three doctors with a hybrid of both in-person and remote visits. She accomplishes an informative encounter by printing out each specialist's visit's SOAP note and distributes them to each professional. By sharing her notes, Leslie reduces in-person treatments by 60%.

2.Mrs. Ella's Case:

An 87-year-old female widow with three middle-aged children, Mrs. Ella, lives alone in rural Texas and was recently diagnosed with a mild form of dementia. Even though she presents no other co-morbidities at this time, she requires monthly consultations with her neurologist and needs a home care representative to come to her house five days a week for eight hours a day.

Her son is a college professor that lives two hours away. Although the other two siblings, also known as supporting primary caregivers, live near Mrs. Ella's home, one works full time and has a family of her own, and the other sibling is herself diagnosed with multiple conditions and is taking care of her sick husband.

Her family found an amazing neurologist who specializes in the treatment of dementia patients and is well-known for his ability to prolong independent living. The physician's philosophy is in line with Mrs. Ella's and her children's primary goal, which is to stay in her house for as long as possible.

Mrs. Ella and her children discussed it, and this is the treatment they want their mom to receive. Because of the limited resources, the uncertainty of this disease, and the location of the neurologist, the primary caregivers will have to reduce in-person neurology appointments as much as possible. At the same time, they have to utilize Mrs. Ella's home care representative's and grandchildren's capabilities to manage virtual medical appointments and trips to the grocery store and other assistance in daily living activities.

3.Adi Johnson's Case

Recently, Adi Johnson, a 19-year-old female with asthma and allergies, moved from her childhood home in South Florida to Connecticut for college. Her pediatrician prepared her for the move with the Patient Better program. Even before Adi moved, she had the contact information for three potential specialists near her college. She anticipates doing more research as soon as she moves so that she can choose whichever specialist she thinks will best match her treatment goals.

Making the most of your virtual appointment

Although privacy is of the utmost importance to all patients, and some might feel uncomfortable with sharing their health information, but, it is essential to have a high-quality virtual visit. If you want a virtual medical appointment to go successfully, you need to be prepared for it in every way. This means being ready to share all information that you or your physician might think is necessary pertaining to your case. It also means that you have suitable audiovisual equipment at your home. Preparation for the virtual visit also means making sure that every gadget and equipment is working as it should. Failing to do so will mean a loss of quality in the visit, and it might also mean the physician might request an in-person visit or maybe a wasted visit due to faulty audiovisual equipment or lack of necessary information.

Use a Quality Camera and set it at eye level so it will be easier to maintain eye contact and stay engaged during the visit. This will allow you to clearly explain your health issues and enable the physician to properly look at your symptoms and health.

Test out your equipment before you start – Make sure the camera/microphone is working properly, and the audio is clear and without static. Ensure that your video quality is not distorted by the light of the window or outside light that may distract the provider but, at the same time, have enough light for clear visibility. Ensure that you are visible and audible and have a translator (if necessary) ready to communicate your health concerns. Plugin your computer or mobile device, if possible, to ensure that your device doesn't die in the middle of your appointment.

Close unnecessary programs - Video streaming takes up a lot of bandwidth, so it is crucial to close all unnecessary programs. Lags in your connection may distort facial expressions and possibly disrupt communication. If possible, use a wired internet connection as it is less prone to interruptions. Also, make sure that you have plenty of power, so your devices won't power-down in the middle of your office visit; remember to plug in your computer or mobile device. Whether you are in a secluded conference room at work or your bedroom, find a quiet and distraction-free space and eliminate potential interferences, disturbances, and interruptions.

2.3 Primary Care Providers: The Modern-Day Medical Concierge

*The complete guide to the modern house call and
concierge medicine through telemedicine technology*

Gone are the days when a medical professional
would come to your home to check on your well-being.
This luxury was known as *"house calls"* and was the
optimal solution for personalized attention. House call
services were delivered in the comfort and convenience
of home and made services accessible to those who were
unable to leave home.

Undoubtedly, when a health professional came to
your home, you were relieved of the stress and the
burden of dressing for the appointment, commuting,
traffic, and waiting with and on others for treatment.
Indeed, a house call removed several inconveniences.
They were simpler days, as there were not the regulations
and bureaucracy that co-exist with today's medical
appointment. But, then again, the chances of you healing
and recovering from a condition have never been so
excellent.

Today, primary care providers offer contemporary
house calls as a service known as *"concierge telemedicine."*
Concierge telemedicine, considered as the new *"house call
of the 1960s,"* is executed when the remote provider and

patient interact in real-time and the entire health history and records are on hand[xxiv]. Unlike urgent care telemedicine, concierge telemedicine providers can follow-up on all the transpired events of the initial diagnosis, offer continual condition treatment, and reduce in-person visits up to 60 percent.

What you need to know prior to establishing a virtual relationship

First, you must commit to your potential concierge provider that you are ready to work a self-management program and understand their potential concerns.

So, what is your primary care provider is concerned about?

- They are afraid of losing you as a patient.
- They are afraid that you may receive too much unfiltered outside unsubstantiated advice, which may affect your ability to follow their treatment plan accordingly.
- They are concerned about ensuring that your health records do not get lost as they are extremely important throughout the treatment.

What you need to do to alleviate their concerns:

✓ State the reasons you are interested in a telemedicine option and let them know that you can handle an equal partnership. Tell them that you are equipped to take care of the administrative duties that co-exist with remote self-health managing.

✓ Do not expect results overnight and stay committed to the complete treatment. If you seek a second opinion, only seek medical advice from a licensed professional and present that information to the doctor if considering any adjustments in the treatment.

Document your health concerns, organize them in your self-health manager, and do not hesitate to share them with your physician if he/she asks for it.

Work needed for concierge medicine

Your primary care physician, with whom you had a face-to-face meeting and an already established relationship. This primary provider has access to your previous medical records. You are collecting and organizing, working with payers, and continuing the long-term relationship with providers. In addition to the ability to perform store-and-forward services, real-time communication, and remote patient monitoring, your primary care physician can perform several services ranging from minor urgent care to long-term chronic condition management all the way to wellness checks and follow-up exams. Let's take a look at what they can be.

The Concierge Telemedicine Uses and Relationship

Just like the in-person office visit the 4 | 6 Step Process should be applied to your virtual appointment (See Article 4.2 in Patient Better: A Comprehensive Guide to Self-Health Management).

- **Chronic condition management** is for patients with long-term conditions at a high risk of being readmitted to the hospital or an emergency room visit.

- **Wellness follow-up exams** are the patients that do not need a full head-to-toe physical examination but need checkups regularly.

- Having a primary provider **helps you reach your goal** of having a familiar face to engage in long-term telemedicine, as well as a continued in-person relationship.

2.4 Specialists

Telemedicine provides patients the ability to be treated by their chosen specialist hundreds of miles away without the need to travel the distance required to see the physician in person

Specialists are doctors who have additional training in medicine that focuses on the prevention, treatment, or maintenance of specific health conditions. These practitioners focus on health issues that need more specialized treatment than what a primary care physician may offer.

Persons with these types of diseases, illnesses, or injuries need exclusive attention at a more in-depth level and are much more likely to end up in the emergency room throughout the occurrence. Statistics show that patients with health issues accounted for 60% of emergency room visits, and of those visits, 30% were most likely preventable[xxv].

For patients who have limited mobility or live in remote areas, telemedicine has become a blessing. It has allowed patients, who typically would not have access to this kind of treatment to manage their illnesses in a more thorough manner. This specific population with complex conditions requires an initial in-person office visit. However, the face-to-face visits are reduced through the comfort level that the patient gains by first conducting regular consultations and medication adjustments then moving to more sophisticated real-time visits. Even though not all office visits can be completed via telemedicine, proper medical care and organized documentation can significantly mitigate your in-person office visits.

Some unforeseen benefits that were brought to the attention of the professionals were that in virtual medical appointments, patients were more relaxed as they were in a familiar environment. This allows the physician to understand specific challenges and patient at-home circumstances more clearly. The virtual medical appointment allowed the physician more closely monitor the patient's environment, provide more individualized patient education, and additional resources if necessary. Real-time appointments also enabled clinicians to offer other more appropriate treatment options when required.

The primary goal when setting up your remote management is to execute effective telemedicine to reducing (1) unnecessary emergency room visits, (2) hospital admissions or re-admissions, and (3) the length of stay. By taking preventative measures of self-managing care. This can be accomplished by having continued interaction and an open door of communication with your specialist, primary care physician, and have an online urgent care contact already in place.

Telemedicine medical appointments available with specialists so far

Neurology

A neurologist is a physician with special training in diagnosing, treating, and managing brain and nervous system disorders. With the patient's detailed medical history, health story, and physical examination, neurologists evaluate the patient's mental status, vision, speech, strength, sensation, coordination, reflexes, and gait.

Common neurological conditions that are qualified for telemedicine include

Alzheimer's Disease - The increasing incidences of dementia in rural areas are in demand and convincingly outweigh its supply. Since the complexes and progression vary from one patient to another, the initial in-person office visit is required. Once diagnosed and evaluated based on the medical history, duration, severity, and symptoms, a treatment plan that includes virtual appointments can be completed, giving the physician more insight into the patient's environment. Continued telemedicine visits, and family participation in self-management, is proven to reduce in-person treatment for this diagnosis by 60 to 70 percent.

Epilepsy - 70% of people with epilepsy can be controlled through medication and routine lab work. Using telemedicine minimizes trips to the office allows specialists to discuss symptom progression and review the diagnostic imaging and blood work.

Multiple Sclerosis - Frequent monitoring of progression is essential for adequately managing this condition and can be done effectively through telemedicine. Medications such as corticosteroids, interferons, and anti-inflammatory drugs may cause serious side effects and changes to the reaction making frequent communication and monitoring necessary. Also, review liver and blood tests can be performed through asynchronous communication.

Neuropathy - Treating neuropathy involves managing symptoms and lifestyle adjustments to help limit progression. Adjusting medication like antidepressants, antiepileptics, and cannabis can be monitored over telemedicine.

Parkinson's disease - Therapies of this condition involves the use of dopamine agonists. In-person rehabilitation is required; neurologists assist therapists through telemedicine to counsel dietary changes, exercise adjustments, and palliative care when needed.

Other telemedicine disciplines and uses

Cardiology - To manage all the plans of treatment for the patients suffering from congenital heart defects and cardiovascular diseases that necessitate ongoing care.

Dermatology - To perform routine skin assessments and triage services.

Endocrinology - To manage patients with conditions such as diabetes and thyroid disease or adjust hormone and hypertension treatments.

Gastroenterology - To treat conditions such as ulcerative colitis, inflammatory bowel syndrome (IBS), or chronic hepatitis C virus.

Hematology/Oncology - To manage treatment plans, medication adjustment(s) for patients who suffer from sickle cell disease, iron deficiencies, and various cancers.

Infectious Disease(s) - To monitor symptom progression, quickly adjust medication levels for antibiotics, antifungals, antivirals, and other treatments in response to unforeseen side-effects.

Nephrology - To manage chronic care or slow the progression of kidney disease, prolong the need for transplants, and create extremely individualized treatment plans for patients receiving kidney replacement therapy.

Pulmonology - To provide treatment for patients with asthma, bronchitis, chronic obstructive pulmonary disease (COPD), and other conditions that require mechanical ventilation.

Urology - To manage the treatment of chronic urinary tract disorders and other complications involving reproductive organs.

Telemedicine for Mental health

The Beginning

Initially, experts did not recognize the correlation between mental and physical health. They were perceived as two separate lines of study of patient wellness. The physical aspect pertained to the tangible diagnosing and treatment of the diseases associated with flesh and bone.

Whereas the patient's mental/emotional and behavioral health dealt with arbitrary conditions that psychiatrists, psychologists, social workers, and counselors focused on. But through consistent investigation experts realized that there may be a correlation between the patient's physical and mental ailments.

Skepticism over the connection between physical and emotional wellness was questionable to such an extent that Dr. Chisolm, the first director-general of the World Health Organization, was viewed as a radical for expressing that psychological wellness care is indivisible from physical wellbeing. He additionally focused on the significance of treating the whole patient for ideal results. This perspective was totally incredible at that point, yet in any case, the idea got on.

To the credit of these revolutionary professionals, people started to realize the inseparable link between physical and mental health. Henceforth, people began to realize the significance of psychiatry, and since then, psychiatry services and developments are accelerating at an extraordinary pace.

Linking Mental Health and Chronic Conditions

Indeed, even as the population of health management programs develop constantly, manufacturing new connections between medical care associations and network administrations, which help patients adapt to depression and anxiety with chronic conditions, still primarily operate with plenty of complications. The guidelines are constantly being developed further and further. Under these guidelines, the primary care providers are motivated to run basic screenings for depression, substance abuse, and interpersonal violence, so these physicians can prescribe appropriate medications and refer patients to telepsychiatry specialists.

2.5 Ancillary Care

Ancillary care is the outside care resources that connect where you live to your chosen health professional

Similar to in-person care ancillary support providers work alongside your primary care provider to aid in treatment and therapy virtually. They not only help with telehealthcare but also behind the scenes in store-and-forward services. Ancillary professionals are a link to patients and specialists as they provide in-person or synchronous treatment and therapy to the patient and then rely on their findings asynchronous to the provider. In this article, we will take a closer look at the healthcare system's ancillary services that are provided outside the doctor's practice.

We will also see how this assistance plays an intricate and essential role in treating and preventing disease and the recovery of your health. Asynchronous technology shines an extremely bright spotlight for healthcare professionals to further understand diagnosis' and execute treatment through *evidence-based medicine*. Asynchronous communication has brought about so many opportunities, is a game-changer for provider-provider communication. Through this channel, providers can more thoroughly assess their patient's use, status, costs, and outcomes and officially record them be examined by another later.

Treat the patient's in-person and asynchronous telecommunication with other professionals

Common store-and-forward services include X-rays, MRIs, photos, and video exam clips. Correspondence fundamentally happens among clinical experts to help in diagnosis. Medical consultations, like live video or face-to-face contact, is not necessary.

Diagnostic imaging and lab tests are used to check a person's health. It is performed in-person, and then the results are read and typically transferred from provider to provider. They can also be followed up with a real-time visit from the patient.

Diagnostic Imaging

Diagnostic imaging is usually performed in a hospital or free-standing facility, depending on its size, location, and specialty. Diagnostic imaging provides clinicians a visual representation of the body's interior health, such as the patient's organs, tissues, bones, joints, and muscles.

Labs

Labs are continuing to extend their services. This includes additional at-home test kits and more. These can be mailed to your home or through a hub-and-spoke clinic. It is an excellent reference for lab testing and where to find them[xxvi].

Doctor(s)-On-Demand

The country's primary care services are also increasing due to a hard deployment of the doctor-on-demand offering. A doctor-on-demand is virtual-care through a telemedicine platform is regarded as temporary primary care offering. Since it's launch doctor-on-demand services developed cross country and has expanded utilization of remote and virtual visits.

Synchronous therapeutic telemedicine services

Physical Therapists, Occupational Therapists, and Speech-Language Pathologists offer telemedicine services as well. There are certain ways you can benefit from telemedicine, but again, knowledge of telecommunicating and self-managing helps in the adaptability of services. Unlike speech pathology, physical and occupational therapy telemedicine is only in the infancy stage of adaptability, and there is much work to be done to refine its patient's embrace. Furthermore, rehabilitative telemedicine in some states is still not universally available to either ancillary service providers or their patients.

Physical Therapy

Rehabilitation and/or physical therapy (PT) are rehabilitative professions that specialize in musculoskeletal conditions and orthopedic and sports injuries. Many patients need essential rehabilitation services, although they are unable to make it to a physical location. It could be for various reasons. For these patients, Physical therapy telemedicine services are good alternates. This way, the patients will get the therapy they need without any physical contact. Also, patients can access quality professional services and education from licensed professionals without even leaving their homes. It also includes post-op patients.

The recovery process can also be accelerated by using various other assistive devices. These are prostheses, orthoses, and the application of heat, cold, electricity, or sound waves. This also enhances the quality of the treatment[xxvii].

Physical therapy

- Pain
- Strength
- Ability to move
- Resilience
- Small and large motor skills (large-muscle movements made with the arms, legs, feet)

Occupational Therapy

Occupational therapy (OT) is the branch of healthcare that enables people of all ages with physical, sensory, or cognitive problems. It enables them to get back their independence in various areas of their lives. Occupational therapists help bring down the barriers that affect patients' emotional, social, and physical needs. They implement various therapies as well as everyday exercises and activities for this purpose. These activities could be getting dressed, bathing, brushing teeth, self-feeding, improving hand-eye coordination, and many others.

The special equipment used for more intervention to regain or build independence include wheelchairs, splints, bathing equipment, dressing devices, and communication aids[xxviii][xxix].

Occupational therapy

- Fine motor skills (small-muscle movements made with hands and fingers for grasping, writing, or typing)
- Visual-perceptual skills
- Cognitive (thinking) skills
- Sensory-processing skills

Virtual Physical and Occupational Therapy work together:

Arthritis	Traumatic injuries: brain/spinal cord	Sensory processing disorders
Chronic pain	Mental health issues	Birth injuries or defects
Stroke	Post-surgical conditions	Learning problems
Brain injury	Burn/Amputation	Autism
Low vision	Severe hand injuries	Behavioral problems
Poor balance	Multiple sclerosis	Developmental delays
Cancer	Transplant	Cerebral Palsy

Pros and Cons of telerehabilitative therapy:

Pros

- Focuses on pain science and patient education.
- Meets today's consumers by delivering on-demand care.

Cons

- Technology cannot provide a therapist's human touch.
- Currently, they are only allowed to treat in the state where they are licensed.
- Lack of multi-state license compact (like they have in PT).
- Patient acquisition is hard enough with traditional clinics; it's even more difficult with teletherapy.
- Spotty reimbursement for services.

SLP (Speech-Language Pathologists)/Audiologists

Audiologists have expertise in forestalling and evaluating hearing and balance issues and give audiological treatment, including listening devices. Speech-language pathologists distinguish, evaluate, and treat discourse and language issues, for example, gulping problems.

Care Alternatives

Retail Clinics

Many retail stores are restructuring their pharmacy and health department to offer people the ability to conduct remote visits with their practitioners through technology. However, the majority of their consumers that need these services are typically an older population. We will touch on this more in chapter three, but in short, these clinics are doing what they can to stay in compliance with Medicare.

Pharmacies

The future of community-centric pharmacies has never been brighter. Local pharmacies that once served as smaller sized general stores, today focus on a more specific health-related product line. While still holding on to their community standing yet think of innovative ways to become even more community-friendly. In most cases, you will find that your local pharmacist and their staff offer medication delivery services, and if possible, offer telemedicine services as well.

They try to provide outstanding customer service and will mostly be on a first-name basis with both you and possibly your provider. For those who value this kind of relationship- this means something- thus positioning themselves to have a leg up on retail chain competitors. People that go to these free-standing pharmacies can bank on having a more in-depth relationship with their pharmacist and receive more individualized services throughout care.

2.6 The Caregiver's Contribution

How caregivers became the backbone in the management of the delivery of at-home care

Family member caregivers have been recently recognized as the most valuable players on one's home care team. These people provide various types of assistance to the patient with their daily living. Clinicians recognize these unpaid and untrained people to provide minimal assistance, but in return, these caregivers stepped up and provided the most qualified and thought-out assistance on the entire home care team.

To distinguish the people who are not compensated and have no formal training, healthcare professionals refer to these people as *informal caregivers*. Informal caregivers are the family, friends, and others in the patient's social circles that help in the injury, illness, or disease. Traditionally caregivers helped their family members in daily activities such as bathing, toileting, dressing, transferring, cooking, eating, medication management, and house upkeep. Today, more sophisticated care is offered by informal caregivers, and if possible, they leave more traditional assistance to home care representatives. The recent transformation of the healthcare clinic, coupled with the upswing of patient's and caregiver's healthcare and condition management knowledge, changed the way professionals view the at-home care team's capabilities.

Now, the challenge lies within the family to manage caregiving with a more structured approach to strengthen the unit's capabilities, to lessen the load for the patient while minimalizing household costs and expenses. In short, people are now expected to think more like a health professional without having prior experience. Informal caregivers must position themselves to see the large picture of an at-home caregiving team and encourages everyone involved in the patient's care to read, participate, and work the activities in the Patient Better program.

Today, health professionals need additional eyes at home.

The Face of a Caregiver

Most caregivers don't consider that they have most likely provided care that significantly impacted the patient's recovery. The simple gesture of driving or medication organization - having experienced people giving care to someone at one point in our life. Informal caregivers are categorized by three stages in life children, adults, and elders. Of those categories in which professionals classify the nurturer and the nurtured: 1) children who are cared for by or are giving care to adults 2) adult children with conditions (that render ongoing assistance) who are cared for by other adults and 3) elders who are cared for by adults (i.e., middle-aged children). The nature of these categories differs.

According to the National Alliance for Caregiving, a 2015 study concluded that 43.5 million Americans cared for another adult or a child with special needs in the previous year. That figure concluded roughly around eighteen percent of the population had help in care from a volunteer caregiver for physical, emotional, and behavioral health.

Demographically, 66 percent of family caregivers are ladies, and astoundingly, 65 percent of care beneficiaries are likewise ladies. The typical caregiver goes through around 20 hours out of every week on providing care obligations.

You rarely find a friend or family who can guide you about the caregiving responsibilities as well as the emotional, physical, psychological, and financial challenges that come with it.

Examples of caregivers

- The fifteen-year-old adolescent was taking care of his mother with multiple sclerosis.
- The foster parent of a 17-year-old girl with Crohn's disease.
- The middle-aged child helping her mother with dementia.
- A father taking care of his child throughout cancer.

- A neighbor driving a friend to Chemo.
- A great-granddaughter coming over to visit her Great-grandmother once a week and playing rummy and making dinner.

A Caregiver's Lot

It is common knowledge that many caregivers often have health issues that they must tend to, along with contributing to another's care. Recognizing that the caregivers' health is most likely compromised, health professionals, realize that caring for the caregiver is just as important as caring for the patient.

When the health professional enters the treatment room, as it is natural to discuss with all that is involved in their patient's at-home care, what they are doing is assessing the total picture and looking for relevant information to help them create the most realistic treatment plan possible. Providers often inspect a variety of potential causes.

These include the patient's and the caregiver's circumstances, capabilities, and limitations. These characteristics are amplified when there is only one caregiver. Individuals and their families living with chronic neurological conditions were caught off-guard when diagnosed. Neurological conditions are not gradual like one would believe; the onset often happens out of the blue. So, in minimal time, families gather, delegate orders, and navigate through the healthcare system. Many health conditions are unforeseeable, and many laypeople do not have the first idea of what to do to manage such conditions and provide the sophisticated care that some diagnosis demand. Individuals as well as families would have thought about the adjustment to their lifestyles, but they have to manage these lifestyle changes now. It can be a very lonely and frightening feeling.

Without knowing, informal caregivers can be detrimental and have a profound impact on their loved one's life.

Even though families know that a time will come when they might have to care for a parent, a spouse, or someone else, they are never ready for it when it actually happens. Taking on the responsibilities to care for a parent can occur during one's life span while raising a family, as a working individual, while chronic condition self-managing, or transitioning care.

Five Benchmarks for caregivers:

- Become educated about the patient's condition-the more you learn about the disease, the more empowered and prepared you are for the role changes.
- Take care of yourself, take care of your family, and practice healthy living.
- Stay social. Learn from others and continue friendships with others and try to remember the past relationship that you had with the one that you are caring for.

- Allow caregiving "holidays" designated to keep your own interests alive.
- Encourage healthy independence of your family, set priorities, and make sacrifices for others. It is a give-and-take type of situation while keeping your own interests at hand[xxx].

Health Effects

Long-term stress and reduced quality of life influence primary caregivers. And the caregiver's health also plays an important role in the patient's well-being. Depression is the second leading condition among caregivers even though many do not seek help. Many families are greatly impacted when coping with their loved ones who have unpredictable conditions. It is impossible to prepare for this kind of onset. Some conditions may last years or decades. Upon knowing this, caregivers' self-care of mental health may be affected. Even as a family, it is a good idea to come together and seek a professional to help walk through the weekly/monthly meetings.

With online capabilities, family members can easily have an informal discussion with the right professionals to help guide them throughout the condition. Caregiving obligation and emotional support run simultaneously with the caregiver's physical and mental health[xxxi xxxii]. It is vital for caregivers to continue with their interests, hobbies, and social circles to supplement and offset the gravity of the strain of caring for another.

Telemedicine Expands the Traditional Caregiver's Self-Managing Capabilities

If you are caring for someone with transitional diseases like Alzheimer's, Parkinson's, or another severe illness or disability, it is likely you have experienced the challenges that come with going to the doctor's office without complication- especially if living in a rural area where access to a specialist is limited[xxxiii]. For most families, when a loved one is diagnosed with a condition, their main goal is to keep all involved in a near-normal lifestyle and not breaking a daily routine. That often includes the patient to live at home for as long as possible, but it also includes the adult children and their children to continue to live in their homes and to worship, work, and attending the same school. More often than not, the extended family joins together and multiple households face the challenges of breaking routines and uprooting schedules, which also puts a strain on the family.

Concierge Medicine On call 24/7

There is nothing more reassuring for the ailing loved one that there is help on call all the time. When the at-home caregiving team builds professional support from licensed professionals, you are combatting against stoke. The home environment is more comfortable and less stress allowing the patient to focus on more important things.

Long-distance Caregiving

Many of us have to care for another over a long-distance. When you are assigned the role of either a clearinghouse or primary caregiver, the first thing that you will want to do is to learn about your family member's condition. This will help you in comprehending what's going on. You will be more prepared to anticipate the next course of action, prevent crises, and assist in self-health management.

Roles may vary, but here are some things that you can accomplish long-distance:

- Assist with finances, bill payment, or money management.
- Arrange for in-home care, contact a social worker, get affiliated with associations that are experts in the medical condition.
- Locate homes to aid in transitional care.
- Provide emotional support.
- Coordinate medical care, research medication, navigate through the labyrinth of new needs.
- Help with insurance claims and processing.
- Keep friends and family informed.
- Spend quality time with your loved one.
- Perform a simple home audit and see if there are arrangements that must be made to relieve other primary caregivers with responsibilities.

Improving Care Coordination

Issues with other informal caregivers and their opinions on how to deliver care can arise. Informal caregivers who take on the role of a power of attorney often have the last say but coordinate with others. Patient Better's Cover Page can be used by all caregivers, both informal and representatives who come to your home.

And, as at-home condition management becomes more complex, informal caregivers continue to take on more roles and responsibilities to aid their loved ones throughout the health occurrence. Patient Better is a unique program as it focuses on the challenges of these informal caregivers to coordinate care, communicate care, and boost health literacy. Being a sole provider also has its own list of challenges. Be open to discussing and brainstorming ways to juggle responsibilities with healthcare professionals and your community. Take direction seriously if the clinician is in touch with an organization that supports caregivers.

Continued Recognition of Caregivers

Recently, researchers have focused on informal caregivers hoping that healthcare may implement strategies to support informal caregiving efforts. There are several challenges to caregivers as they must coordinate care across multiple social and healthcare organizations and obtain access to needed services.

Informal caregivers are the newly recognized heroes of the United States healthcare system. And at some point in our lives, we will all become informal caregivers. Even though they are vital to patients, these caregivers go unpaid and without formal training.

Although there is no remedy for such a time to juggle strenuous responsibilities and work, There are more organizations on the horizon that can develop skills as a caregiver. Upon delivering care for a loved one, it is important for you to cognitively take care of yourself as well. Professionals now recognize that caregivers do their best to avoid burnout. The list below are some ideas of what people have done, and you might want to consider implementing into your life to help better take care of another.

2.7 Urgent Care, On-Demand, and Behavioral Health Services

The after hour go-to for on-demand medical services

Urgent care specialists, doctors-on-demand, and behavioral health professionals can supply and are the most familiar virtual services. These services are convenient for everyone who travels extensively, need care in the middle of the night, or just prefer staying home, these telemedicine services are just a ping away.

Urgent care

People living with chronic conditions are three times more likely to end up in the emergency room than healthy individuals. Urgent care telemedicine services are unique as they can help guide you in the direction of what to do right now and further evaluate whether an emergency room visit is absolutely necessary.

To receive an optimal urgent care experience, research should be completed long before an urgent care consultation is conducted. Some considerations, for various reasons, should be recognized prior to calling an urgent care specialist. Your chosen urgent care is to have an actual physical location of an urgent care facility along with their in-house telemedicine services. An established relationship will add cohesion so that you can immediately get in touch with someone with just a couple of swipes or strokes of a couple of keys.

You don't need a caregiver who might say, *"I'm debating on going to the emergency room,"* or *"Could you let me know if we can handle this through video conferencing or make a physical appointment?"* You must use your better judgment. However, if you are uncertain, and your urgent care specialist recommends in-person treatment- be ready to move, call 911 or go to the nearest clinic.

Doctor-on-demand

These primary medical services are provided as an alternative or an addition to concierge services. Doctors' on-demand services are rendered when patients are not able to see their primary care provider. Like urgent care telemedicine, the doctor's on-demand services are typically available 24/7 and will help with short-term medical care or until you can visit your primary provider.

But don't think about replacing your concierge provider with a doctor on-demand as they cannot follow-up appointments or supply long-term services like treatment planning, etc. For various reasons, such as location and medical availability (i.e., not having access to the internet), or the patient is immobile and does not render emergency care, on-demand services are a less expensive way to correct health issues before they get out of hand.

Although popular, doctors on demand can still offer limited services; they will get you where you need to go or to the next step until your next meeting with your primary provider.

Behavioral Health

Studies have found that chronic physical conditions, mental and emotional conditions go hand in hand. People living with chronic physical conditions often experience emotional stress and chronic pain, which results in depression and anxiety[xxxiv].

Take the example of diabetes, where the condition is known to disrupt blood circulation and fluctuate blood sugar levels that impact brain function as well. One of the results is distress and isolation from social support. The evidence clearly suggests that depending on the severity of the symptoms of the chronic conditions, the patient will experience more mental health issues. Therefore, it does not come as a big surprise that people who suffer from chronic physical conditions are often those who report poor mental and emotional health.

Mental and physical conditions can also have many of the same symptoms like decreased energy levels, fatigue, and food cravings, thus contributing to weight gain. This makes the individual more prone to other mental conditions. Behavior telemedicine has the potential to be the key to supplying the emotional care needed by people who live with chronic illness[xxxv]. Collaborative mental healthcare initiatives link primary providers with mental health specialists to offer support for people who live with poor mental conditions.

Behavior health for caregivers

Many unpredictable neurological conditions such as multiple sclerosis, Alzheimer's disease, Parkinson's disease, Huntington's disease, or stroke have long durations that affect the caregivers' emotional state. And as the disease progresses, the increasing symptoms create the need for family members to provide more extensive care.

Family members have to take care of the patient and take care of the finances, household, and more. This impacts the caregiver's mental health along with their ability to continue providing care. These responsibilities often fall on the immediate family member's shoulders, such as the spouse or child(ren).

Caregivers are also prone to a considerable increase in their own physical and psychological symptoms during caregiving. Some diseases do not shorten the lifespan but complicate it. Thus, the role of at-home caregivers can extend for many decades. As the patient's physical, emotional, and cognitive needs increase, the less time the caregiver has to devote to their own needs, their family member's needs, home life, and career. The significant demand for caregiving takes a toll on the caregiver's endurance and coping mechanisms[xxxvi].

Section Three:
Telemedicine Preparation

This chapter focuses on what's behind telemedicine laws, regulations, and policies allowing people to see the full picture of the office visit. Through this chapter's insight, you will build the inner skills needed to show the professionals how serious you are in becoming a partner in care.

Key Takeaways

Improve self-discipline- Formulating a routine of preparedness and develop good habits that co-exist with successful telemedicine.

Enhance strategic thinking- Removing the stressors that often come when discussing health information with a professional online. At times you need to complete the more complex task of strategic thinking (remotely) and be ready for unpredictable health events.

Develop resilience- Is the ability to think positively throughout the entire health journey. This may be an incredible request for some, but it is important for yourself and the ones who care for you for an easier health experience.

3.1 The Fine Print in Telemedicine

Connecting medical services to federal and state requirements, insurance guidelines, and patient compliance

Twenty percent of Americans with chronic conditions live in rural areas, whereas only nine percent of specialty health services are delivered[xxxvii]. Many believe that telemedicine may be the answer to help connect these rural Americans (with limited access to care) to the specialty care that they need. It is speculated that telemedicine may also be the answer to reduce unnecessary spending, further accessibility, and increase the physician's and the patient's ability to monitor chronic conditions more closely.

The demand for specialized care in rural America is highly desired. In summary, one source stated that "Among eleven industrialized countries, the United States ranks the lowest on the measurement of care in regard to efficiency, accessibility, and equality[xxxviii]." As it stands today, the American Telehealth Association is the only known organization that completely focuses on accelerating the adoption of telemedicine.

"As it pertains to telemedicine: advocating and bettering patient-centered services; patient-provider communications; patient self-management with provider feedback; health

literacy; medication management; provider-provider consultants; and changes in health and lifestyle behavior[xxxix]*."*

Concerns of Telemedicine Implementation

Some healthcare professionals are concerned that their patients may not acclimate to the offered virtual services. They are also worried about their patients' adoption capabilities. The future of funding and support for telemedicine after the pandemic is yet to remain seen. Some believe that if patients are not responsible to care for themselves after an in-person consultation, then surely their level of interest will drastically decrease with virtual appointments. We will go on to discuss this in detail later, but as it stands today, the common belief is that virtual communication remains more challenging than interacting face-to-face.

Simplifying Complexities

For healthcare provider's and insurer's virtual healthcare concerns, for the most part, are the same as in-person concerns, with one difference: the distance. Telemedicine should benefit the patients, the providers, and insurers alike – as all three contributors have some sort of benefit in telecommunication.

As it pertains to healthcare professionals, they need to benefit from their expanded services. They need to make sure that it is right fit for their practice. But as far as reimbursement is concerned, telemedicine service fees not as straightforward as traditional in-person medical services for one reason, the lack of patient data to support the encounter. For various reasons, patients are not providing their vitals which limits the physician's ability to empirically treat and document medical necessity to insurers.

Standardizing Telemedicine

The Federation of State Medical Boards (FSMB) is an organization that guides physicians in licensing, disciplines, and regulations. The FSMB set the standard that telemedicine services must adhere to and recognized to the same standards as in-person services. When technology and healthcare collided itself into fruition, [at the time] it made the experts realize the optimal solution for virtual encounters would be to equalize real-time visits to the already structured in-person appointment. Since parity law was already established, it made it easy to formulate telemedicine guidelines around the already rooted regulatory and administrative requirements[xl].

Healthcare's Parity Laws Explained

Within the world of telemedicine, a parity law is defined as the diagnosis and treatment of patients in remote areas transmitted over distances through telecommunication.

Parity

In short, *parity* means equal.

Law

The word law refers to the set of rules and principles entrenched in a community by respective authorities as applicable to its society and enforced by a judicial decision whether in the form of legislation or of customs and policies; laws are recognized.

Healthcare's parity laws pertain to both face-to-face encounters as well as telemedicine services. The idea behind structuring healthcare laws in this manner is to recognize that both in-person and virtual services are the same (or equivalent) to traditional medicine delivered inside the doctor's office and must meet the same documentation requirements as well.

Healthcare Parity Law Is Broken Down into Federal and State Guidelines

1. State parity laws, which are laws in healthcare that rest on the state level in which practitioners must deliver services with the same standards of virtual medical care as in-person care services. Medicaid and private insurance companies are expected to reimburse virtual healthcare professionals the same as in-person service providers.

   This standard also includes medical necessity determinations by physicians, and the criteria of the individual health plans must be equivalent. Services must be reasonable, necessary, and appropriate. And like in-person visits, your plan coverage approval is the same and the reason for private payer coverage denials are available upon request.

2. Federal parity laws are laws in which the federal insurer, Medicare, sets guidelines in which they commit to follow and display them on a public forum in an effort to lead by example.

About Federal Healthcare Parity Law

In 2012, with the Affordable Care Act in action, the federal government made its first move to encourage telemedicine services to be included in coverage. These remote services were implemented only for under select circumstances at the federal level through Medicare. However, Medicaid, on the other hand, remained within the powers of the individual states.

Here is a list of guiding principles for federal policy:

- Reduce and remove barriers to telemedicine, including geographic discrimination and restrictions for managed care
- Prevent new barriers, such as rules that force higher-quality standards for telemedicine as compared to in-person care
- Encourage the use of telemedicine to reduce health delivery issues – such as provider shortages.
- Enhance consumer choice- better outcomes, provide convenience, and increase satisfaction.

Medicare's Evolving Telemedicine Offerings

Medicare's telemedicine services were offered to patients who lived in rural areas. The idea was that the specialist provided satellite offices in outlined areas with a connection to their main practice. The benefit to the patient is that they only had to travel to this minimally scaled office nearest to their home. The satellite office had the communication equipment in place and lower-level medical assistant to usher in, check vitals, and connect the patient to the practitioner. This form of synchronous communication is referred to as hub-and-spoke.

However, on 6th March 2020, in the wake of the COVID-19 scourge, Medicare agreed to pay for telemedicine services without the previous hub-and-spoke restrictions. It means that while the pandemic emergency is going on, most, if not all, Medicare patients will have access to in-network telemedicine services in a real-time remote setting. In other words, the patient is no longer required to travel to a satellite office. A telemedicine visit can be conducted in the comfort of home and Medicare will reimburse the clinician.

Healthcare Parity Laws on the State Level

The policy landscape from state-to-state is continuously in a condition of flux. There is always a juggle to balance laws and policies regarding reimbursement through state programs and commercial payers. State laws govern commercial payer's policies. Ostensibly, the implementation and use of telemedicine vary from state to state regarding what services providers will be reimbursed for.

The state, likewise, governs what kind of "parity," characterized as "equal treatment of services," is normal between in-person health services reimbursements and telemedicine reimbursements. This variety influences suppliers' capacity to actualize telemedicine choices, hence decreasing these services.

This doesn't help patients become less confused or more at-ease with telemedicine processes. As a result, telemedicine faces considerable obstacles in becoming accepted by patients to expand the doctor's office's offerings. Until then, states and the nation cannot fully realize the cost-effectiveness of telemedicine.

Each state has developed its own telemedicine parity laws, which means that along with Medicaid, commercial and private payers must also follow state telemedicine guidelines.

Equal benefits

If a plan must follow federal parity law, these treatment limits and payment amounts must be covered equally:

- Inpatient in- and out-of-network services
- Outpatient in- and out-of-network services
- Partial hospitalization
- Residential treatment
- Emergency care

- Prescription drugs
- Co-pays
- Deductibles
- Facility types
- Provider reimbursement rates
- Clinical criteria used to approve care

The State and Federal Fine Print

Suppose there is an established parity law in a state as compared to an already secured federal parity law. In that case, it means that the private health insurance plan must follow state regulations as the federal parity may only make inclusion for optional benefits. Federal parity may replace state law only when the state law "hinders the application" of federal requisitions. For instance, if state law demands coverage for certain health conditions, then the federal requirement of equal coverage will surpass the weaker state law[xli].

Connecting the Dots...

After the healthcare professional's services meet the standard of federal and/or state regulations and insurance plan(s), they are ready to offer telemedicine services. If the adoption of recently lifted telemedicine regulations is followed appropriately, the belief is that even though some services may be implemented, others may not. Like in-person services, a review must be completed for each encounter. If the vitals are not properly documented on the telemedicine visit, just like the in-person visit- the encounter may be determined by insurers that the encounter is incomplete. Therefore, it is imperative for patients to understand and follow guidelines and keep up to date of insurer's requirements.

Insurance Guidelines

Under the 1135 (Coronavirus) waiver the location of the patient and provider (as long as they are in the same state) and the location of the remote session is irrelevant. Under normal circumstances and the state of emergency is lifted, all the same guidelines of insurance reimbursement approval remain in a virtual appointment as it does an in-person encounter. However, when this particular waiver is reinstated, it may be that the virtual appointment will not be reimbursed. It may be that insurances may go back to previously recognized guidelines and hub-and-spoke synchronous communication may be reinstated. I mention this because this is something to keep an eye on after we get back to "normal".

3.2 Financing

Connecting federal and state policies, weighing Medicare, commercial insurance, and cash-pay options for both in-person and virtual office visits

Virtual medicine is quickly entering mainstream medicine as a practical and relatively inexpensive tool to render medical services at a distance. It will not be long before telemedicine acceptance grows, services expand, and protocols mature.

Instrumental Self-Managing Components

The principal overseer (clearinghouse) of your self-management system determines why the telemedicine visit is conducted and what is to be accomplished. I have created a Patient Better SOAP Note and Treatment Plan Calculator that is dedicated to documenting telemedicine encounters. Clearinghouses can utilize these worksheets to help guide primary and secondary caregivers to outline the virtual appointment to review later. Projection of the costs for the visit coupled with document management, the responsibility of governing in-person and virtual appointments will also fall on the clearinghouse's shoulders. The bottom line is that healthcare professionals are in dire need of patients and family-member caregivers to play a more active role in care, not only in the delivery but also in the management of documents and administration[xlii]. Having an at-home support team participating in a self-management program is the solution.

Direct Healthcare Costs

As it stands today, most healthcare spending encompasses in-person medical encounters which are more than any other developed nation.[xliii] The US spends nearly three trillion on healthcare every year. And of this spending, an estimated $200 billion of that spending is avoidable[xliv] simply by catching: (1) the side effects from medication early and (2) physician's knowledge of their patient's non-compliance. Telemedicine can mitigate a good share of these expenditures just by simply supplying access to instant and continuous healthcare. The lifted restriction gave people a glimpse of what telemedicine can really do. Real-time visits give people a connection to healthcare like never before. Now, it is up to the patients to fulfill a deemed completed encounter by providing the necessary information that insurers require.

Indirect Healthcare Costs

As discussed in Patient Better: A Comprehensive Guide to Self-Health Management, indirect costs include vehicle wear and tear, gas, parking, time off work, child or adult care, and other schedule interruptions. On the premise that telemedicine can reduce in-person office visits, it is believed that telemedicine curtails the total indirect patient costs.

Telemedicine's Financial Responsibility Upgrades

In the past, providers were seldom reimbursed for providing incomplete telemedicine consultations. And resultantly, virtual medicine was brought to a halt and it struggled to gain traction. This has historically been a barrier for providers to implement and impacted their willingness to adapt telemedicine. However, the pandemic and has rapidly changed the professional's enthusiasm to embrace synchronous communication for the better. As a result, the patient's and their caregiver's views of remote medicine revitalized itself as a more trustworthy system.

The joining of self-management and equal partnership will also include another expansion of responsibilities in financial management. With new self-managing competence, people become more efficient in financial managing. Taking self-managing from strictly in-person scenarios to upgrading visits in telemedicine, the expectation for laypeople to organize in-person and virtual insurance claims and well as cash pay. With confidence, self-managers can examine the financial document in question and explain concerns with the adjuster, biller or social worker who is best suited to answer queries in a timelier manner. Patients who have this kind of responsibility for financial management, including tracking expenditures and understanding the basics to protect themselves from fraudulent claims.

Lifted Medicare Restrictions Provided Unforeseen Opportunity

Traditionally, Medicare has only reimbursed for store-and-forward and hub-and-spoke communications and did not reimburse for in-home real-time services. Many restrictions applied to the services that the insurance covered. While under the COVID pandemic the Centers for Medicare and Medicaid Services (CMS) for a limited time removed the hub-and-spoke mandate and agreed to provide real-time telemedicine services remotely. This initiative was taken under the patronage of President Trump. This means that many beneficiaries are now able to receive better care for a broader range of services from healthcare providers in the comfort of home and additional effort to shelter-in-place. Under this waiver, a wider range of services is now being offered to patients. This waiver and the flexibility is all about containing the spread of the virus and keeping as many people as safe as possible.

As the spread of the pandemic is still not in control, and there is uncertainty about the situation, telemedicine is the need of the hour. The people who need regular and routine care but are vulnerable can now benefit from this service without the need to leave their homes. Concomitantly, telemedicine will maintain the access to the care in which the underserved are so desperately in need, reducing the exposure to help slow the spread.

Commercial Insurance Follows Suit

In the last decade, third party payers like Cigna, United Healthcare, Blue Cross Blue Shield, and Medicare have been working tirelessly to expand telemedicine services. Due to tremendous cost-savings, better patient results, and being immensely helpful to the patient (and family), insurance companies realize that telemedicine just makes sense.

The pandemic has temporarily removed existing obstacles a crossed many insurers. Leaving only state parity laws to be followed for reimbursement, the patient must reside in the same state and have an existing in-person relationship with their virtual physician. So, on top of short-term temporary care services people have the opportunity for long-term chronic condition management. Because of the constant transformation, it is always best to double-check with the insurer for the details about whether they cover telemedicine and whether they will cover services from any particular licensed professional.

What would be the cost?

If your insurance company does not offer telemedicine reimbursement in your state and you and your doctor agree that telemedicine services are suited for you, you and your physician can sign an agreement to waive insurance and go with cash pay.

More Access to Care

Insurers and regulators are looking for new ways to mold state parity laws to accommodate the new evolving traveling patient. Cross-state licensing would do is that as it'll allow health professionals to provide care to a patient in any nigh state without acquiring a full license to practice there. Several states are working to pass measures to allow state medical boards to establish cross-state licensing.

If you have two or more treatment options

- Measure the length of time it would take you to meet your projected goal.
- Calculate the projected total costs
- Evaluate the most relevant treatment that you feel you will be most successful in completing.

Under the 1135 Waiver Starting March 6, 2020, the office and hospital visits furnished via telemedicine are coverable by CMS and also include the patient's place of residence. Patients will have access to doctors, nurses, psychologists, and licensed clinical social workers, among others.

Additionally, the HHS Office of Inspector General (OIG) provides affability for healthcare providers to curtail or relinquish cost-sharing for telemedicine visits paid by federal healthcare programs. All Medicare patients will be able to communicate with their healthcare providers using the patients' portals without going to the office.

Key Takeaways

- Virtual services can be provided if you already have an established relationship with the licensed professional.

- Under the 1135 waiver, limited coverage does not only apply to persons living in rural settings or approved hub and spoke locations.

- Individual services need to be agreed upon, and your provider may educate you of the services before the agreement.

- If your known physician, employer, or health insurance plan offers telemedicine services, then your decision to choose a virtual provider becomes easier.

- Registration and a secure internet connection are all you need to set a telemedicine appointment under commercial and federal payers (for now).

- As the costs covered by your existing payment methods might not be consistent with coverage under telemedicine- check with your insurance company for updates.

3.3 Creating a Google Health Account

Know how to organize your care for virtual medicine, provide a resource hub of communication, and join your entire care team in real-time at a distance

Google is Patient Better's recommended online health account for various reasons. It is an online platform that connects the provider's electronic recording system to your Self-Health Managing system for both real-time and store-and-forward communication.

The functionality, versatility, security, and accessibility are the primary components that make Google a good hybrid-fit for managing dual healthcare systems. The principal reason for choosing Google is that it applies uniformity and supplies privacy like no other platform. It is the number one resource that supplies a variety of tools for individuals to communicate with others. Google is available on both iOS and Android mobile devices and tablets as well as Windows, Mac, or Linksys computers.

Many of you already have a good understanding of how to manage your standard and non-standard health information in your Self-Health Manager, now we will create an extension online. Patient Better's "Google Health Account" is created for you and your family to enhance health communication, use, status, reduce costs, and better outcomes. Although I have created a video on

YouTube, I still encourage you to read this article so you understand why it is important to create an account with Google.

If you are the Clearinghouse, then the primary responsibility for Google setup would be yours. Still, if you are unfamiliar with the Internet, then you can collaborate with another primary caregiver. Setting up and understanding Google is essential in organizing your telecare. When you get the chance, please review and see Patient Better's YouTube videos.

Here is what a Google healthcare account supplies

Accessibility- Google's secure platform is recognized by most doctor's offices' electronic health records as well as your at-home caregiving team. It is easy to obtain and use, and easily accessible.

Security- A Google healthcare account can supply adequate security measures to protect your private health information and adhere to HIPAA compliance measures.

Functionality - It is the quality of serving a purpose well; A Google healthcare account offers a range of operations that enable you to run your account properly and communicate with other electronic systems.

Versatility- Google can integrate with various other platforms. This versatility allows you to adapt to many different health dynamics and family situations.

Google Chrome

Google Chrome is a browser used to access the internet and to run web-based applications. This means that you will be able to bookmark and make history searches for everyone involved in your care.

Benefits: Bookmarks and settings synchronization

Chrome is feature-rich and enables its users to synchronize their bookmarks, history, and settings across multiple devices that have the browser installed by sending and receiving data through the chosen Google account, which updates all signed-in instances of Chrome.

Google Gmail (email)

Google email or Gmail is an email service offered by Google that is free. Users can access Gmail easily on the web as well as use third-party programs to synchronize email content through POP or IMAP protocols. Gmail started as a limited beta release on April 1, 2004.

Benefits of Gmail: Real-time instant messaging and secure video conferencing

The benefits of this email service are that it has a huge storage space. You can have online access anywhere. It is cheap and doesn't need a lot of maintenance. It has synchronization capabilities, stores instant messaging and video conferencing, and easy search and organization tools to hold all of your Contacts. It also provides security for data.

Google G-Suite

Google G-Suite is a suite of tools, software, and products developed by Google related to cloud computing, productivity, and collaboration It was first launched on August 28, 2006, like Google apps. Those apps can create an email specifically for healthcare, online storage, calendar sharing, video meetings, and more. The G Suite also provides access to several powerful Google applications, including calendar, docs, sheets, slides, forms, pictures, and Hangouts.

Benefits of Google Apps: Making Communication and Collaboration Simple and Effective

By using Google apps, you can easily share all your documents, conduct video conferences, and use instant messaging within your email. You can also invite others to share your calendar, making at-home caregiver meetings and doctor's appointments easy to plan.

Suggested Google G-suit Apps

Relatively inexpensive, free for most, but the paid version could make it more robust with additional extensions that could incorporate all caregivers' schedules.

.

Google Search Engine- Let's Google it! Google is Patient Better's optimal search engine to locate any desired health research. It provides user-friendly, simple, and targeted results. Users will be happy when they like the search results that Google delivers based on their search queries. The answer is simple: happy users turn into repeat users and repeat users turn into loyal customers.

Calendar- Put the Google Calendar on all your devices and share it with others. You can also synchronize it with other smartphones and tablets and connect them to other caregivers. This integrated online shareable calendar designed for teams can keep routines, schedules, and health and intellectual activities. It allows you to share someone else's plan while creating your own events and sharing them with your teams. This keeps the entire team connected.

Hangouts- Utilize this app for video and group messaging and keeping in touch with long-distance clearinghouses, healthcare professionals, and primary and secondary caregivers for a unified communication service. This will allow everyone on the care team to text, voice, and video chat in either a one-on-one setting or a caregiving group.

Drive- Google Drive is a cloud storage system that enables users to store all their files on Google's servers, synchronize them across multiple devices, and easily share them with others. It was launched on April 24, 2012. In addition to that, Google Drive also offers apps with offline capabilities for Windows and Mac OS computers and Android and iOS smartphones and tablets. This parent app unites, synchronizes, and organizes child apps such as documents, spreadsheets, pictures, drawings to communicate all of your health issues with your entire at-home care team.

3.4 Interpreting Medical Notes

Reading and interpreting standard medical notes for a more robust health story

Patient Better defines standard medical notes as recordings created by licensed healthcare professionals to document an encounter for the purpose of assessing, evaluating, measuring, and predicting care of the individual's wellness or occurrence. As your self-managing skills develop

In Patient Better: A Comprehensive Guide to Self-Health Management, we discussed financial statements and standard in section three. Then we connected the non-standard records in section four. Then we concluded how to create non-standard notes and forecast and measure conditions in section five. Similar to non-standard healthcare documents, standard medical notes are the optimal way to asynchronously communicate with everyone on the care team.

One Patient, Two Forms of Records

1. Standard Medical Note

A standard medical note is an entry created by a licensed professional to document their patient's history, diagnosis, treatment, or progress. Four out of five healthcare professionals write standard medical notes in the SOAP note format. Ideally, clinicians write notes accurately and in their entirety. In these documents, providers include all relevant information of any given medical event that cover diseases, major and minor illness or injury, and the continuity of care. Healthcare providers have electronic health records that safeguard these notes and alerts clinicians of any missing, incomplete, or inconsistent data.

The anatomy of a standard medical note will include seven characteristics that certifies that it is an official note: (1) the title of the document that is appropriate of the circumstance. (2) the practitioner and the medical facility in which the clinician practices. (3) the date that the document was written. (4) the patient's name and other related information such as age, gender date of birth. (5) the purpose of the encounter. (6) the certification of the condition which is where the clinician specifies illness, injury, and condition of the patient and (7) a summary of the plan. the person who wrote the document's signature[xlv].

Four Examples of Standard Medical Notes

1. The Summary Note

A medical summary is a restatement from a licensed healthcare professional of the conversation and findings during your encounter. Although the summary does not typically include a diagnosis, the medical summary note may consist of your medical facts, health history, current well-being, and the expected medical condition in the future.

When creating a medical summary, clinicians examine the completeness of your records. They extract relevant information that includes test results and other treatment histories and apply it to your current standing and ability to perform daily tasks such as work, fitness, and social activities. This document also details any medical conditions, complaints, medications, and how they developed over time.

An example of how a patient may use a medical summary note

The patient went to an orthopedic expert to discuss a hip replacement. The patient's visit and symptoms are described in the summary. The doctor discussed the future steps with the patient. These steps included further follow-up appointments that the patient will have to come to. The patient used that summary to keep reminders about those appointments. Additionally, the patient also showed the summary to a family member so that they can help him with the care and saved the note in his self-health manager communication pocket to review and analyze in case he wants to get a second opinion.

2. The Progress Note

A progress note is a report that details the patient's clinical status or achievements during hospitalization or outpatient care.

An example of how a patient may use a progress note

This patient is going through depression and anxiety and has weekly virtual therapy sessions with a mental health professional. Recently, the issues became worse due to a diagnosis of Parkinson's disease. The therapist described in detail the patient's emotional and physical symptoms and also discussed some coping strategies in the therapy session. He also made a progress note of it all.

When the patient received the progress note, she was relieved to know that the therapist completely understood her condition. Since Parkinson's disease affects memory, she can now depend on the progress notes to remember what she needs to do in between office visits. Additionally, the patient will bring this progress note and her self-manager to the physicians that prescribe medications so that all members of her healthcare team can be informed about her care.

3. The Condition Management Note

A condition management note acts as a structured treatment plan that aims to help you better manage health conditions and provide information to maintain or improve your quality of life. A condition management note may include the goal of improving your long-term condition. Conditions such as asthma or diabetes require regular monitoring to prevent progression. A condition management note is essential to both improving outcomes and containing costs.

An example of how a patient may use a condition management note

The patient suffers from multiple health conditions including type-II diabetes. He has to take several medications at a time and utilizes his notes to manage his health as well as his medications. He remembered a time when he was on an out-of-state business trip, and he forgot his medication. He called in for a prescription and picked it up from the (nation-wide retail) pharmacy but realized that his dose appeared incorrect. He was able to look over his latest condition management note on his smartphone and correct the issue after business hours.

Additionally, he receives care at one hospital but his endocrinologist is located at some other hospital, but he can print his notes and store them in his self-health manager to bring this correction to the other physician's attention involved in his care. He has a busy schedule to juggle and finds it extremely important that all of his information is accessible by his entire health team. He feels more like an expert in his condition since he caught the potential error and says that he feels healthy, even though he has a complex medical life.

4. The Pre-Surgical Note

This medical note is a pre-operative assessment of your medical history, current health status, and home circumstances. This note also considers any medical problems that may need to be treated before surgery and if any special care after surgery is required.

An example of how a patient may use a pre-surgical note:

This patient required a throat operation, and her otolaryngologist needed to determine if she could be fitted with a breathing tube during the surgery. The surgeon summarized her medical history and described the examination that was performed. The note contained some complicated terminology, for example, otorrhea and more that the patient could not comprehend. She was able to look up the terms online and write a list of questions to prepare for surgery. She also shared the note with her primary provider in a different hospital affiliation.

Non-Standard documentation

Non-standard documents are recordings from people that do not have a license to practice medicine and are not formally trained in the specified area. The individuals who write these notes cannot be recognized in a court of law. Non-standard notes are important and can be an extremely informative communication tool throughout the entire care team. Your spiral notebook (health journal) and worksheets are provided so that you and other caregivers can write non-standard information about your health and care. It is important to consistently update your journal as there is a cognitive and emotional connection associated with reflecting your health on paper in real-time. Descriptive writing about your healing journey helps facilitate growth, understanding, and insight into your illness.

Writing also helps improve mental clarity, solves problems, and sustains overall focus. Any other small issue of concern, you can note as if a family member has a health issue that may be hereditary. Jot down everything and anything that you want to and be as detailed and specific as possible. Caregivers should be motivated to keep a log journal. Your notebook is the primary personal health record, and the Patient Better templates summarize your entries and can serve as shorter versions for clinicians.

2. Non- Standard Medical Note

A non-standard note is a recording of the patient's health at any given point of care outside the professional environment. Although helpful for healthcare professionals for patients to write long versions in SOAP note format, 80-90% of non-standard notes are written with only one to three sentences and later to be interpreted and vetted by clinicians in case further investigation is needed. It is important that the clearinghouse organizes the documents in the Self-Health Manager as well.

Review questions to ask yourself when reading standard medical notes

- Are the medications, symptoms, and health conditions accurate?
- Does the information in the note reflect what was discussed during the visit?
- Is this information something that I want to share with my other health professionals or at-home caregiving team?
- Is there anything that I need to clarify?
- Is there anything that I don't understand that may require research or professional clarity, such as medical terms, a diagnosis, or treatment recommendations?
- Is there any information, like symptoms or family history, that I forgot to share during my appointment?
- Are there any inaccuracies in my note that should be fixed?

How to Manage Medical Notes

The clearinghouse has access to all standard and non-standard notes and is responsible to double-check notes and detect discrepancies and inaccuracies for standard notes and petition the creator (doctor, nurse, physician assistant) for an amendment if necessary. As well as check for inconsistencies from contributors to avoid a lapse or inconsistencies in at-home care.

For every document inside the Self-Health Manager, the clearinghouse examines and coordinates both standard and non-standard records between all care providers to reduce duplication of medical services or oversight and reap the benefits of better care coordination. Indeed, a note, if not organized correctly, poses a greater risk of being lost, devalued, and interpreted as a *loose note*.

Section Four:
Actively Teleself-managing Care

Preparing for your telemedicine appointment is the next step toward having a significant, purposeful virtual encounter with your healthcare professional- every time. Practical application of self-management for in-person and virtual medical appointments. Greater purpose to cognitively fit into the telemedicine market as an active participant as a patient and as a desperately necessary component to make healthcare better.

Key takeaways

- Make a lifelong commitment to adapting to new healthcare delivery models.
- Strategize and individualize telemedicine visits with providers to receive equivalent virtual visits to in-person appointments.

4.1 The Modern Provider-Patient Relationship: An Equal Partnership in Care

Self-managing care transitions the patient-provider relationship from the traditional provider-patient model to an equal partnership in care

In the previous chapters, we examined the traditional provider-patient relationship and how and why we must transform it into a partnership. Through examination, we were able to conceptualize the immediate need for us to form this partnership for the betterment of our in-person and virtual office appointments. Now, it's time to actively move our familiar relationship into an Equal Partnership in Care (EPIC).

Some health care professionals may argue that there is no concrete reason to change the traditional behavior of the provider-patient relationship. Indeed, if those clinicians prefer the hierarchal relationship as it stands, and they feel that a face-to-face visit with their patient is better. This argument may hold true in some cases, and if the doctor prefers this kind of relationship, it is best to follow each clinician's guidance[xlvi]. However, in other cases, when the health professional is familiar with self-management and the patients and their family-member caregivers need to take advantage of telemedicine's benefits, then, the equal partnership in the care model is optimal. With self-management you and your entire at-home care team should be able to seamlessly juggle each professional's preferred provider-patient relationship style.

The EPIC concept advocates that patients should actively participate in the health care services they receive. Hospitals developed the EPIC concept in the understanding that the patient and family-member caregivers are considered as full-fledged partners on the care team. This way, the patients' and caregivers' experiences and knowledge are recognized.

The Patients as Partners concept was developed by the Faculty of Medicine at the University of Montreal and its affiliated hospitals. They conducted a study to better understand how the patients and their family view their engagement with health care professionals regarding their care. In this study, the patients appeared to play a more active and less docile role in their direct care, as suggested under the processes of learning, knowledge, and adaptation. Whereas the researchers had a clarity of the processes' benefits when they broke them down for further investigation: (1) that the learning process allows patients to acquire experiential learning about their health and technical information. (2) the knowledge process involves the patient's ability to assess and understand the care that they had received, their experience, and how it aligns with their own personal preferences. (3) the adaptation process involves the patient adapting to the healthcare service, which was built on the patient's learning and assessments, concluding their ability to adapt and what has been perceived as optimal or non-optimal circumstances. This assessment also included the quality of the patient's relationship with their health care professional as a partner[xlvii].

The Complex Diagnosis and the Equal Partnership in Care

Providers are thoroughly trained in the patient-provider dialogue and understand the ways of discussing the diagnosis. The physician anticipates a shift in the patient's sense of self and is trained to handle this information exchange and what comes afterward (i.e., tests and treatment). This is an important part of the encounter and continued partnership.

Self-managing each appointment

Self-managing care is a new concept for most. However, many of us, with the help and guidance of our physicians, have created a self-managing system for as long as we have been going to the doctor's office. All Patient Better did was form a structure to your existing self-management capabilities. Self-managing is an amalgamation of you and your professional's governance of care. And the move from a relationship to a partnership greatly depends on the comfortability of the people who self-manage care. As a layperson you may have professional questions that need to be answered by your clinician, in the same way, don't hesitate to reach out to your professional to help in determining which appointments require an in-person or remote encounter. Office visits are completed from appointment to appointment meaning that once the first appointment is conducted then at the conclusion of that appointment you and your healthcare professional will determine if the next appointment can be held remotely or face-to-face.

Be inquisitive

The term health literacy has been coined by the professionals to describe the patient's ability to find out, analyze, and comprehend the basic health information about the services needed to make appropriate health decisions. Health literacy directly affects healthcare service delivery, including healthcare costs, healthcare use, healthcare status, and healthcare outcomes. Inside every skilled "self-manager" is someone who is proficient in health literacy and the importance of being inquisitive.

Inquisitive Communication

Being inquisitive while at the doctor's office visit is healthy. Prepare your questions in advance so that your questions present themselves with more validity. Also, if something comes to mind, speak up, and elaborate if necessary. This will ensure that you receive a quality education from your trusted and licensed professional and that you won't have to do it alone.

Here are some examples of questions

- What preventative care services are right for me?
- Are there any online resources I can trust for medical information regarding _____?
- How does my family medical history affect the risk for _____?
- Why is this medication being prescribed?
- Will flying after surgery affect my recovery?
- How could (insert condition) affect my health down the road?
- Does my lifestyle such as (five-hour sleep regimen) impact my health?
- What do you do for your personal wellness?
- Does my child really need (an antibiotic) for this or do you have alternate suggestions?
- My real fear is _____. How concerned should I be?
- Can we talk about end-of-life care?[xlviii]

Your Relationship with Your Insurers (Keeping a good document trail)

The primary benefits of knowing how to work with your insurance company is that you can find and fix errors on your medical statements and safeguard yourself from financial errors. This gives you more control over your care. Keeping a good document trail just like the professionals provides a heap of benefits to you. With time, it becomes easy to implement and manage. You increase your productivity and eliminate human error as well as reduce unnecessary costs[xlix]. Furthermore, your satisfaction level with your health care will improve as well as your ability to maintain compliance.

Children, Medical Management, and the Professional Partnership

A study has shown that physician-patient-parent communication indicated that the physician's communication with children 10 and younger was predominantly ineffective. However, the clinician's communication with the child's guardian was predominantly instrumental[1].

Naturally, parents take care of economic needs and serve as an authority figure to help make decisions within a family. The trick is for the parent to observe when the child is ready to self-manage care and relinquish their established responsibilities and transfer them to the child.

Children who learn about self-managing care early in life through participation in clinical encounters develop communication and decision-making skills from the very start. This sets the stage for an experience that enhances communication between the young adult and the provider. When teenagers begin to develop more self-identifiable information than their parents, individual participation reduces complications, improves self-advocacy skills, and the overall satisfaction of the young patient's healthcare experience.

The Impact of the EPIC Relationship for In-Person and Virtual Medical Appointment

Patients of all ages and at-home caregivers will have access to remote care. Primary examples of users in need of virtual care are:

1) Those who travel extensively.
2) Those who have debilitating conditions that prevent them from leaving their home.
3) Those who live in rural areas with limited access to care.
4) Those who are in desperate need of telemedicine services in a continuum for care.
5) Caregivers who care for others with complex health conditions (and maybe who are immunocompromised themselves).

These folks will reap the benefits of managing their care more efficiently: staying independent longer and heightening their family's ability to deliver care more efficiently.

4.2 Telemedicine Appointments

The virtual visit has the same processes and protocols and should be treated equal to an in-person appointment

Preparing for your virtual appointment will give you the ability to think things through more thoroughly in an online environment, and better evaluate scenarios. In this article, Patient Better helps you develop a formula for synchronous communication preparation.

Create Identical In-Person and Virtual Medical Office Appointments

Your Google or "G-Suite" health account is a way for you to organize and communicate electronically with both physicians and family members about your health. Your G-Suite creation is a single informational hub that stores records, allowing caregivers access to important updates and documents in real-time and asynchronous communication. Among the many simplified, patient-friendly benefits, you will have the ability to transfer protected information that falls under HIPAA compliant guidelines. Also, your G-Suite account improves your experience of organizing and making remote healthcare easier.

Your Self-Health Manager is a hard copy for in-person medical office visits that aid in places where online access is not always available. And your Self-Health Manager is an assistant to help you throughout both your remote and face-to-face sessions. You can turn your Self-Health Manager into a chronological guide of your health journey to help walk you through each appointment or to regroup with other at-home caregivers.

Set the Scene

The online appointment should be conducted in a quiet, private place (away from children, pets, and other distractions). Make sure you are ready ten to fifteen minutes prior to the appointment. You'll likely talk to an assistant for a pre-assessment, and then be connected to the physician for the professional evaluation. Most appointments last about 20 to 30 minutes. Ensure that the phone or computer's battery is charged and have your health management tools in front of you. Have a pen and paper handy. Gather all related medical equipment such as the thermometer, inhaler, and other devices and equipment if appropriate. If you use an app or electronic device like a peak flow meter to track symptoms daily, have it close at hand. It turns out that many telemedicine appointments fail because of a simple reason such as battery failure or distractions like family or children at play.

Make sure you are in an area with good cellphone reception. If you're using FaceTime, Skype, or Hangouts, or any other application with video, give it a try before the visit starts. Make a dummy call to a friend or relative to check the quality. That way, you can troubleshoot and remove any obstacles.

The Office for Civil Rights, the organization that enforces HIPAA, has stated that telemedicine should not be conducted through Facebook live, TikTok, or other public communication services

Plan your approach

Think about what you want to accomplish during the visit. Your goal could be to understand your medications or treatment options, renew a prescription, get training about a specific medical condition, or a Q and A session to better understand symptoms and side effects. You could have multiple goals during your office visit as well, and in those cases, try to prioritize what's most important for you during the encounter.

Just like an in-person visit, telemedicine appointments will have you talk with a nurse or medical assistant for a pre-assessment before connecting you to the physician. Keep all information in the Self-Health Manager.

Equipping yourself with the necessities:

✓ Chief complaints are written in your SOAP note

✓ Document vitals 30 minutes prior to appointment: blood pressure, weight, heart rate, and temperature.
✓ Medical history, including current and past onsets, conditions, and surgeries.
✓ Prescriptions and over-the-counter medications, herbal supplements you use (including vitamins and natural remedies).
✓ Your pharmacy's phone number and address.
✓ (If seeing a specialist) Your primary physician's name and contact info.
✓ Insurance information or credit card for payment.

Equipment

✓ **A computer or smartphone-** that has two-way video conferencing capabilities along with a camera and speakers.

✓ **A thermometer-** to check your temperature. A thermometer will inform you if you are feverish or not. It is advisable that you check your temperature orally if you are experiencing body aches or chills. For babies who cannot keep the thermometer in their mouths or there is the risk of them breaking the thermometer with their teeth, check rectally. Forehead and armpit readings tend to be inaccurate and should be completely avoided. A fever is defined as 100.4 degrees Fahrenheit or above[li].

✓ **A blood pressure monitor-** A blood pressure cuff can help you ensure any medication you take for hypertension is doing the job accurately. Your blood pressure objective relies upon your age and medical conditions, so ensure you ask your primary care physician what number you need to focus on.

✓ **A camera-** to take a picture, and if your appointment is a couple of days away, you may want to take multiple pictures. Remember to put the date on each one.

✓ **A scale-** to verify your weight. You will be able to assist the doctor in detecting your weight at the same time every day and keeping a record. This is especially true if you suffer from a condition like heart failure that causes you to retain fluid in your body.

✓ **Other devices-** that may be pertinent to your condition. This could be a glucometer to help people with diabetes keep tabs on their blood sugar levels. If you've been told to use one, track your values so you can discuss those with your doctor during your tele-visit.

Paperwork

- ✓ Telemedicine SOAP Note
- ✓ Latest medical note from the previous visit
- ✓ Insurance ID
- ✓ Driver's License
- ✓ Patient Better Forms

Communicators

- ✓ Internet connection

✓ Email
✓ Communication system (Clinic's portal, Facetime or Zoom)
✓ Have your Google health account and Gmail address available and your portal connected to your provider's health system

Finance

✓ Check and verify insurance and understand what charges are associated with the appointment.
✓ Have a credit card ready for payment (co-pay, deductible, or full cash pay)

Once the visit is done, most of the telehealth providers will send patients an email regarding patient assessments and instructions. But, it is still advisable to take notes and then comparing them with the email so that you understand everything clearly.

The challenges of telemedicine

Our goal as patients is to support this technological form of medical service delivery. Meticulous preparation and proper self-management for any medical appointment are necessary these days. Like the in-person office visit, the medical staff prepares a treatment room specifically for you, free from distractions.

You must set a similar scene for your telemedicine appointment. You must create a quiet place where you can focus — a place where you would feel comfortable in openly engaging with your provider. Like the clinician, you must have any and all notes, reports, and documents ready and your Self-Health Manager within an arm's reach. Like the provider, you must take your appointment seriously. Afterall, what would you do if you went for an appointment and your doctor was distracted or ill-prepared? You would feel extremely frustrated over the loss of time. The same is true for the doctor, too. I can't stress this enough; telemedicine is in the wild-west phase of implementation. We are all working to provide structure for telemedicine, and all three groups (providers, payers, and patients) are interconnected, all mutually benefiting each other. If one fails to perform, then no one in the group will be able to satisfy the other group's demands.

Make sure that you have your vitals checked 30 minutes before the appointment. Be ready to report your findings at the very beginning of the appointment. Use specifics when detailing your health concern(s). For example, if you have a low-grade fever for three days and it spiked to 101.6 in the last day that prompted you to make a telemedicine appointment, make sure you are ready to state your fever's history and verbalize each individual condition. "My (1) fever is like this, (2) coughing began when X, (3) my runny nose developed after X".

Each chief complaint should include these five elements:

1. **Primary Mention** - When did the health issue start?
2. **Location** - Where is the issue located?
3. **Duration** - How long has the issue been going on?
4. **Severity** - How bothersome or disruptive is the issue?
5. **Secondary Mention** - Why did the health issue start?

Self-Health Manage Your Way to Better Virtual Care

Going back to the 4|6 Steps of the Medical Office Process (See Patient Better: A Comprehensive Guide to Self-Health Management Article 4.2) diagrams are equivalent for virtual appointments as it is for in-person visits. Make sure that you follow all of the rules of this process and be prepared to support each process accordingly (Patient Better: A Comprehensive Guide to Self-Health Management Article 4.2).

Like the in-person office visit, you can expect a 20 minutes face-to-face virtual visit with the clinician. This might seem like a long time, but you will want to complete the pre-work before the actual consultation to get the most out of the examination as possible.

Answer the provider's questions as clearly and to the point as possible

Just like in-person office visits, be prepared to answer the value-based practice routine questions:

1. How is my patient doing today?
2. How will my patient respond to our treatment or therapy?
3. What will the impact be on my patient over time?

As in the S.O.A.P. Note format, you can expect your virtual appointment to be processed similarly.

Device and Medication Compliance Records

Have your device(s) ready (upon request) for the physician that prescribed the device along with your report of compliance or use. If you are not using the device as recommended, share that with your provider. It would allow them to understand your compliance issue, and they may come up with an alternative solution. Always request a report of the visit after every appointment. Make sure that your email address is up to date and provide that in every office visit. Medical notes are written notes created by a licensed healthcare professional and can be used as a formal document to provide you with comprehensive recommendations and assist you in preventing, maintaining, and treating medical issues. Label your notes accordingly as a summary, progress, condition management, or pre-surgical.

If possible, you want to get the most out of your appointment and skip the trip to the physical office. If you are ill-prepared and the provider cannot properly treat you remotely, then they may require you to come in. Ultimately, it's up to you to make telemedicine work.

4.3 Self-Management, Your EPIC Relationship & the Myths and Truths About Telemedicine

Appointment preparation and self-health management skills to build and maintain EPIC relationships

Over the last decade, telemedicine has slowly and gradually moved into the space of functionality. Now telecommunication must focus on the adaptability of persons with more sophisticated medical issues. The healthcare needs of America's deserving patients with chronic conditions can be successfully fulfilled with telecommunication. However, many consumers remain skeptical due to its lack of (believed) availability. This is a considerable barrier that telemedicine's implementers must focus on extinguishing.

What I have observed is that consumers are concerned whether their telemedicine services are covered by insurance or not. As a result, the solution would be for insurers to better help their patients understand their plan. Another way the professionals could help patients increase adoption is to structure a patient-centric telemedicine platform. I believe that telemedicine can be made more mainstream and better accepted by patients with complex conditions if they were provided with proper guidance other than a quick one or two lined advertisement, which in my opinion; is simply not enough. It wouldn't be enough for me or my family, anyway. At the core of all telemedicine challenges, as telemedicine has been an uphill battle ever since its conception and the lack of proper implementation lies, not only in telemedicine's go-to market strategy, it also in the patient's ability (or inability) to self-manage care. Which is the primary reason of why I wrote this book.

To explain, for years, providers and insurance companies have tried to make telemedicine work, but they left you — the patient — out of the equation. Why? Because there is an underlying belief [among providers and insurers] that patients don't want to [or know how to] contribute to the improvement of healthcare. But the solution to their concern is simple, and it's something that we [patients] all must do as recipients of care. The missing component for patients to participate in self-management is key to help in the improvement of healthcare. Laypeople must take an active role in self-managing.

For remote healthcare to work properly, telemedicine needs a united trio of equal partnerships of providers, insurers, and patients who are willing to do what it takes to make telemedicine work. In Article 4.1 The Modern Provider-Patient Relationship: An Equal Partnership in Care we formulated the immediate need to implement the EPIC Partnership, on the larger scale, there is also a great need to develop this kind of ownership of responsibilities. So in essence, each interconnected group can fulfill one another's primary desired goals: 1) providers want to offer quality services equivalent to in-person treatment, 2) insurers want cost-efficiency and want to know that they are being reimbursed for the same quality services as in-person visits, and 3) patients want convenience and continued accessibility to care. All three must operate together in an interconnected, equal partnership for telemedicine to work[lii].

The bottom line is, if patients do not self-manage care properly, then providers will not be able to execute a thorough telemedicine consultation and therefore must leave a lot of necessary information out. And if there is missing information, then insurance companies will not feel comfortable reimbursing for an incomplete service, and vice versa. If an insurance company does not feel comfortable reimbursing for remote medicine, then physicians are compelled to hold in-person office visits.

Before providers and insurance companies can feel comfortable adding patients into a telemedicine partnership, you must first transform your traditional patient-provider relationship. Change it from a paternal, hierarchical interaction into an equal partnership in care, and be ready to transform your patient-centered care into a relationship-centered care model if necessary. (For more detail, please see Patient Better: A Comprehensive Guide to Self-Health Management Part 4, Article 1).

Once healthcare professionals feel comfortable with your medical record management capabilities and your preparation and participation in virtual office visits, and your insurance company is confident that you are keeping a good document trail, then they will embrace you as a team player and work with you on a professional level. With the third group (of patients) joining into the mix and contributing to telemedicine's functionalities, remote healthcare services will overcome its implementation challenges.

Working behind the scenes, telemedicine unites and builds on these new working relationships so that all three key players can get what they want: 1) providers can deliver a complete and comprehensive virtual service equivalent to an in-person office visit, 2) insurance companies can comfortably reimburse accordingly and 3) patients can self-manage their conditions more easily and continue to get access to remote care.

Myth #1: Telemedicine is just an on-demand service for people who have concerns about conditions like the flu, a rash, or a runny nose.

Truth: People might think that telemedicine is just for basic care services due to the virtual nature of a video-based care visit. While telemedicine is commonly used to provide urgent, care–like services, the reality is that concierge telemedicine services include follow-ups, post-ops, and long-term maintenance care. Telemedicine is expanding its available services every day. For more comprehensive consultations and services, patients must learn to self-manage care.

**Myth #2: Only those with computer skills will do
well in virtual visits.**

Truth: Once you are comfortably self-managing care,
the transformation from in-person to virtual medicine
will become less confusing, and your primary provider
will become your concierge physician. Your first video
conferencing appointment may have hiccups. Proper
preparation, video technology, and a secure and reliable
internet connection is a must. And rest assured, the other
person on the phone (or computer) completely
understands your predicament and is ready and skilled
to help you along the way. You may want to bring your
laptop, smartphone, or any other handheld device to your
next in-person visit and ask a staff member to download
or set-up their portal on the device.

**Myth #3: Telemedicine does not protect health
information.**

Truth: Two-way communicators such as Skype,
Facetime, or Hangouts are safe and effective tools that are
deemed as "compliant" to complete a reimbursable
telemedicine appointment. Whereas public platforms
such as Facebook, Instagram are not. Make sure that you
are in a quiet location where you can openly discuss your
health. The security algorithms for these apps are
continuously being updated, and your information will
be safe.

Myth #4: Virtual medicine is less expensive than an in-person medical office visit because it's less effective.

Truth: Telemedicine physician costs are reduced because their overhead costs are reduced, including limits to inventory costs and equipment sterilization needs. Operating costs such as electricity, staff, insurance, mortgage payments, and other costs associated with having a brick-and-mortar location are also reduced.

Myth #5 A physical exam is not necessary before a concierge telemedicine consultation.

Truth: In cases where your health condition initially presents as a skin rash, congestion, or a mild fever, a doctor on demand can treat your ailment. However, suppose your care requires long-term attention, such as follow-up visits, regularly scheduled maintenance, or post-op visits. In that case, your primary physician will require access to your complete medical history and, in those instances, an in-person exam before concierge medical service.

Myth #6: Telemedicine technology cannot provide the same intimate relationship as an in-person office visit, and the at-home caregiving team may find self-managing care challenging.

Truth: Once an equal partnership in care is created and the relationship-centered care model is established within your team, then you can rest assured that everyone on your at-home care team and all your health professionals will be on the same page.

Myth #7: Doctors cannot conduct a thorough examination through telemedicine.

Truth: In the early days, telemedicine was primarily a phone-based interaction between a patient and a provider. As smartphone technology has evolved, so has virtual medicine. The providers' ability to conduct real-time video visits has created a far more intimate interaction between the patient and the provider. Virtual visits stand a greater risk of being incomplete as physicians are unable to access key vitals such as temperature, blood pressure, or body scan images. However, this obstacle is changing—and fast. As home-device makers are creating incredible, yet very reasonably priced technologies, where a physician will have access to the desired health information, and the patient can utilize the device in their home. Patients who complete the pre-work before the remote visit greatly enhance the provider's ability to examine, access, diagnose, and treat. This enables the physicians to perform more robust consultations and more thorough evaluations and expand the healthcare services that can be delivered at home.

Myth #8: Telemedicine is complicated, confusing, and overwhelming to learn; a trip to the doctor's office for an in-person examination is sufficient.

Truth: For most adults where mobility is not an issue, going to the physician's office is not a challenge. But for people who are disabled, extremely sick, bedridden, or suffering from some other illness that doesn't allow them to move freely, telemedicine might be their only option for a high-quality consultation[liii][liv][lv].

4.4 The Future of Telemedicine, Further Adaptation, and Conclusion

Building a foundation and a continued partnership of self-management and telemedicine to meet the needs of today's health consumer's demands

The Need of the Hour

If implemented properly, telemedicine can be perceived as a fruit tree that will keep on producing food for decades to come. As the tree matures, the stronger and more resilient it becomes. The benefits of proper self-management and telemedicine capabilities usefulness today and what future lies have yet to be known.

Telemedicine bridges the gap between patients, physicians, and insurers. Virtual medicine enables everyone, including patients and the ones who care for them, to stay at home and communicate with physicians through reliable and state of the art technology. Telemedicine has really stepped up to the plate during our recent pandemic and is now emerging as a viable tool for precaution, prevention, and treatment[lvi]. However, it remains to be seen how it will impact those who need it the most after the COVID pandemic subsides.

Before the pandemic, only 26 states were reimbursing healthcare professional services for consultations. This is based on payer policies and state laws. For the most part, clinicians are looking for a less expensive way to deliver care that is most effective, most convenient, and can offer the patient the highest value. At this point in time, telemedicine seems to be the answer.

Telemedicine programs seem to be appearing everywhere, with employers offering services to their employees, healthcare systems implementing programs, and national telemedicine providers creating standalone offerings. Seventy-seven percent of users said that they would be more likely to choose a healthcare provider who provided telemedicine as compared to a physician who did not use technology. Also, there has been a seven hundred percent increase in the number of telemedicine consultations. Interestingly enough, just eighteen percent have used telemedicine services, and it has yet to become the standard for care.

Patients seek out healthcare experiences similar to their experiences in other industries in terms of ease of access and instantaneous answers. Telemedicine service providers are structuring their programs to provide this ease and instant answers to patients and their family caregivers.

Telemedicine programs are better equipped to address today's health consumers' support needs. They can do that in such a way that traditional telemedicine care just cannot without self-management. For this purpose, the first thing that the organizations have to understand is what individual patients demand apart from the basic needs for quality care and a good experience. This could be a long-term partnership in the continuum of care throughout the patient's life irrespective of where they are located at.

Patients do not want to be sick or spend considerable time finding the care to remedy their illness. People who are outside of the industry want the least number of disruptions and distractions throughout their daily lives, regardless if they are sick or injured. The lifestyle of many patients makes accessing care less about priority and makes it more challenging to comply. For example, (1) an individual who is suffering from a chronic illness needs follow-up appointments but cannot do so because of a demanding job and family requirements will often put themselves last. (2) A caregiver might want to be present at a loved one's medical appointment but cannot do so because of family obligations and lack of understanding of the seriousness of their loved one's ailment. (3) An individual goes through with surgery but cannot make it to the follow-up appointments as they don't have the time or find it a priority to go to the physician's office if they feel better.

So, keeping in view all the above, telemedicine can be viewed as so much more than an on-demand urgent care appointment. It is an integrated component of the care continuum. Telemedicine is an opportunity to meet individuals where they're at, regardless of whether that is at the home, office, school, or another area, to guarantee they're getting the care that they need. Eventually keeping people well or making it simpler for them to get well with negligible disturbance to their day-to-day life.

This implies that remaining healthy is not a burden but accommodates the modern-day's health consumer's way of life.

Telemedicine and Self-Health Managing Fosters Relationship-Centered Care

For organizations that don't have a wide variety of telemedicine services, assessing where to begin offering Telemedicine or how to expand the offering should be looked at in a patient-centered fashion. A few examples of patient-centered telemedicine services include:

- Telemedicine intensive care units allow patients to stay close to home and receive higher levels of care without being transferred to another facility This is especially valuable in rural settings.

- Remote patient monitoring allows patients to record critical health information and share it with physicians so they can monitor their conditions more closely without a formal appointment.

- Virtual sleep studies performed at home offer minimal disruption to daily routines and enable those who can't be away from home to undergo this test.

- New moms can now access lactation consultations via secure mobile apps and overcome any challenges that they face with breastfeeding. They can get the guidance and assistance no matter the location.

Today, the array of telemedicine's innovative ideas can go on and on. But that doesn't mean every organization must offer services. It is important to talk to your doctor about the need for virtual medicine. What their goals and objectives are in their practice to truly understand what's preventing patients from complying with physician recommendations such as returning follow-up care, completing a recommended protocol, or even seeking out care when they are well. Telemedicine is beneficial for patients by designing a treatment plan that better meets a patient's lifestyle, but it will be increasingly important as physicians take on risk.

Telemedicine is very likely to stick around. Studies prove that more than 55% of patients reported a satisfactory experience while using telemedicine[lvii]. And healthcare professionals believe telemedicine use will increase.

There will be some adaptation barriers, but the target audience must be considered to determine who would fit the best for telemedicine services (this will probably be everyone). At the same time, you want to connect to the folks who need it the most. The ones who live in rural areas are unable to find transport from one place to the next. Telemedicine is attractive, but most people don't know where to begin and don't think about reading up on it until they fall sick. But by then, it's too difficult to put in the research needed to make telemedicine worthwhile on your own.

Even though more and more commercial insurers are now covering telemedicine services, the level of adoption is still very low. This is because of Medicare as they are slow in increasing the offers to patients who are outside of rural areas. Even though a compelling argument could be made for physicians to adopt telemedicine, healthcare insurers have always resisted the idea of paying for the technology involved.

This is due to the fact that it has made bold claims about reducing the cost. Consider this scenario. A $50 telemedicine video visit to diagnose an ear infection is much cheaper than a $2500 trip to an emergency department. The same is true for elderly patients who suffer from multiple chronic conditions. But telemedicine didn't have much of a track record admittedly when it went public. Telemedicine was relatively new and unproven. It was uncertain whether it would achieve and sustain high demand for the patient and family member caregivers' acceptance and market adaptation. Payers fear that telemedicine will just become another add-on to the services that already are being provided. Think of a phone call or a Skype chat before or after the official visit.

"Medicare, in particular, has been afraid telemedicine will blow the doors off of spending," says John Linkous, CEO of the American Telemedicine Association.

In 2020, all the skeptics' cost concerns are being legitimately handled by the introduction of higher quality video equipment, access to smartphones, and higher, faster Internet connections. Clearer, sharper telemedicine interactions presumably will prevent patients and family member caregivers from making duplicative in-person medical office visits.

As more people come to value telemedicine, and better documentation of the encounter come to fruition, it's likely insurance will recognize that telemedicine visits are equal to an in-person visit and will continue coverage. States are moving quickly to establish their standards and continue reimbursement after this pandemic.

Glossary

*4|6 Step Medical Process: Patient Better's explanation of the healthcare practice's and patient's series of steps and actions needed to take to complete a successful medical office visit

Activities of Daily Living (ADLs): A term used to collectively describe fundamental skills that are required to independently care for one's self. These activities include keeping a safe environment, bathing, breathing, communicating, dressing, drinking, eating, eliminating, and sleeping.

Asynchronous telecommunication: patient information that is transmitted between healthcare professionals to send electronic reports, results, and other medical-related data to be reviewed by the receiver at a later time.

*Clearinghouse: Refers to a primary caregiver or patient that is considered the leader or overseer of the Patient Better Program. Takes on the primary responsibilities and delegates tasks needed within the home of the patient.

Document Management System (DMS): A technological system in which healthcare clinics implement into their practice to track, manage, and store documents. Often related to electronic record management system.

Electronic Health Record (EHR): This is a patient's medical record that is stored electronically within a protected health entity.

Electronic Medical Record (EMR): This is a patient's medical record that is stored electronically in private practices.

Health history: In clinical medicine, the patient's past and present that may lead and contain relevant information bearing on their health past, present, and future. The medical history comes up as an account of all medical events and occurrences that a person may have experienced, and this is an important tool in the management of the patient.

*Health story: Chronological personal remembrance of one's life or health occurrence that may include emotions, pain scales, status, reactions, circumstance, and underlying events and causes.

Health Insurance Portability and Accountability Act (HIPAA): A United States law that designed privacy standards to protect patients' medical records and other health information provided to healthcare professionals, medical offices and hospitals, and third-party payers.

Hub-and-spoke: The hub-and-spoke is synchronous communication that is applied in healthcare settings. Hub-and-spoke is a method of organization involving the establishment of a main campus, or hub, and is complemented by satellite campuses or spoke

*Informal Caregiver: Are people (typically family members) who have taken on the responsibility to care for another that go unpaid and have no formal medical training that helps the patient with daily living activities.

*Loose note: This is a note that does not pertain to any specific project or relevancy structure or arrangement.

Meaningful Learning: (ML) refers to the concept that previously learned knowledge is fully understood by the individual and that the individual knows how that specific information relates to other stored data (stored in your brain that is) and is applied to the newly learned material. For understanding this concept, it is good to contrast meaningful learning with the much less desirable, rote learning.

Meaningful Use: Meaningful Use means that electronic health record technology is used in a "meaningful" way and ensures that health information is shared and exchanged to improve patient care. According to the CDC, there are five "pillars" of health outcomes that support the concept:

Meaningful Use:

- Improving quality, safety, and efficiency while reducing health disparities
- Engaging patients and families
- Improving care coordination
- Improve public health
- Ensure privacy for personal health information[lviii]

Medical Record: This is a compilation of written or digital notes, documents, reports, observations, and patient information created by licensed healthcare professionals to record a specific health occurrence and treatment. Medical records are then submitted and stored within a medical entity's database to be reviewed for an extended period of time.

Patient-Centered Care: Involves individual patients in their specific care demands. The IOM (Institute of Medicine) defines patient-centered care as: "Providing care that is respectful of, and responsive to, individual patient preferences, needs and values, and ensuring that patient values guide all clinical decisions."

Patient Engagement: "Patient engagement" is a broader concept that combines patient activation with interventions designed to increase activation and promote positive patient behavior, such as obtaining preventive care or exercising regularly.

*Primary caregiver: A primary caregiver is someone who's faced with the duty of taking care of a friend or loved one who is no longer able to care for themselves. Primary caregivers may be caring for children, a senior, a spouse with a terminal illness, or any friend or family member who requires assistance with daily activities.

Relationship-Centered Care (RCC): is a framework for conceptualizing healthcare that recognizes that the nature and quality of relationships in health care influence the process and outcomes of health care. An extension of Patient-Centered Care, Relationship-Centered Care is founded upon four principles: (1) that relationships in health care ought to include the personhood of the participants, (2) that affect emotions are important components of these relationships, (3) that all health care relationships occur in the context of reciprocal influence, and (4) that the formation and maintenance of relationships in care participation are morally valuable[lix].

Remote Patient Monitoring: Remote patient monitoring is a technology to enable monitoring of patients outside of conventional clinical settings, such as in the home or in a remote area, which may increase access to care and decrease healthcare delivery costs.

Retail Health Clinic: A retail health clinic is a walk-in clinic located in a retail store, supermarket, or pharmacy to treat uncomplicated illness and provide preventative healthcare services.

Self-management program: A self-managing program refers to a program that helps people who have ongoing health conditions and caregivers learn how to manage their care more effectively. For many people, a self-managing program reduces stress, allowing them to follow treatment more closely and identify financial errors, duplicate tests, and become more proficient in health communication and literacy. Self-management education programs are clinically proven to reduce symptoms and improve quality of life.

Synchronous telecommunication: Real-time communication conducted by the provider and patient to exchange information in a live setting.

Telehealth*: Telehealth is the distribution of health-related services and information via electronic information and telecommunication technologies primarily used among health professionals Includes learning, continued education, through means of virtual technology.

*Telemedicine: the remote diagnosis and treatment of patients by means of telecommunications technology. It allows long-distance patient and clinician contact, care, advice, reminders, education, intervention, monitoring, and remote admissions.

*Secondary Caregiver: are trained to assist the elderly, disabled, mentally ill, and/or terminally ill. **Home care** assistants often work in private **homes** to help patients with daily tasks such as personal grooming and meal preparation

Store-and-forward: Store-and-forward telemedicine is collecting clinical information and sending it electronically to another site for evaluation. Information typically includes demographic data, medical history, documents such as laboratory reports, and images, video and/or audio files.

Virtual Medicine: The term virtual medicine refers to the treatment of various medical conditions long-distance through means of telecommunication. Telemedicine platforms include live video and audio, instant messaging in a remote setting.

* Denotes a unique Patient Better definition (medical jargon) may have multiple meanings in various settings

References

[i] Stefano Omboni, Luca Campolo & Edoardo Panzeri (2020) Telehealth in
  chronic disease management and the role of the Internet-of-Medical Things: the Tholomeus® experience, Expert Review of Medical Devices, 17:7, 659-670, DOI: 10.1080/17434440.2020.1782734

[ii] Holman, H., & Lorig, K. (2000). Patients as partners in managing chronic disease. Partnership is a prerequisite for effective and efficient health care. *BMJ (Clinical research ed.), 320*(7234), 526–527. https://doi.org/10.1136/bmj.320.7234.526

[iii] Bashshur, R. L., Shannon, G. W., Smith, B. R., Alverson, D. C., Antoniotti, N., Barsan, W. G., Bashshur, N., Brown, E. M., Coye, M. J., Doarn, C. R., Ferguson, S., Grigsby, J., Krupinski, E. A., Kvedar, J. C., Linkous, J., Merrell, R. C., Nesbitt, T., Poropatich, R., Rheuban, K. S., Sanders, J. H., … Yellowlees, P. (2014). The empirical foundations of telemedicine interventions for chronic disease management. *Telemedicine journal and e-health : the official journal of the American Telemedicine Association, 20*(9), 769–800. https://doi.org/10.1089/tmj.2014.9981

[iv] Pearson, Elsa, and Austin Frakt. "Administrative Costs and Health Information Technology." *JAMA Health Forum*, JAMA Network, 3 July 2018, jamanetwork.com/channels/health-forum/fullarticle/2760147.

[v] Heath, S. (2020, November 19). Why Patient Education is Vital for Engagement, Better Outcomes. https://patientengagementhit.com/news/why-patient-education-is-vital-for-engagement-better-outcomes.

[vi]"Health History." *Encyclopedia of Surgery,* www.surgeryencyclopedia.com/Fi-La/Health-History.html.

[vii] Bae J. M. (2015). Value-based medicine: concepts and application. *Epidemiology and health, 37,* e2015014. https://doi.org/10.4178/epih/e2015014

[viii] NurseJournal.org. (2020, December 2). *Tips to Improve Patient Education.* NurseJournal. https://nursejournal.org/articles/tips-to-improve-patient-education/.

[ix] Paterick, T. E., Patel, N., Tajik, A. J., & Chandrasekaran, K. (2017). Improving health outcomes through patient education and partnerships with patients. *Proceedings (Baylor University. Medical Center), 30(1),* 112–113. https://doi.org/10.1080/08998280.2017.11929552

[x] Paterick, T. E., Patel, N., Tajik, A. J., & Chandrasekaran, K. (2017). Improving health outcomes through patient education and partnerships with patients. *Proceedings (Baylor University. Medical Center), 30(1),* 112–113. https://doi.org/10.1080/08998280.2017.11929552

[xi] "Why Is Self-Management Support Important?" *AHRQ,* Agency for Healthcare Research and Quality, Rockville, MD., 2016, www.ahrq.gov/ncepcr/tools/self-mgmt/why.html.

[xii] Kyle, S, and Shaw, D. "Doctor–Patient Communication, Patient Knowledge and Health Literacy: How Difficult Can It All Be?" *The Bulletin of the Royal College of Surgeons of England,* 12 June 2015, publishing.rcseng.ac.uk/doi/abs/10.1308/rcsbull.2014.96.6.e9.

xiii N. (2015, August 17). *10 Benefits of a Document Management System in Healthcare*. Polar Imaging. https://polarimaging.ca/10-benefits-of-a-document-management-system-in-healthcare/.

xiv Koren, Daniella. "The Impact of Knowledge: Patient Education Improves Compliance and Outcomes." *The Wellness Network*, 4 Oct. 2016, www.thewellnessnetwork.net/health-news-and-insights/blog/the-impact-of-knowledge-patient-education-improves-compliance-and-outcomes/.

xv Catalyst, N. E. J. M. (2018, February 1). *What Is Telehealth?* NEJM Catalyst. https://catalyst.nejm.org/doi/full/10.1056/CAT.18.0268.

xvi "About Telehealth Store-and-Forward (Asynchronous)." *Thumbnail*, 2020, www.cchpca.org/about/about-telehealth/store-and-forward-asynchronous.

xvii "What Is Telemedicine?" *VSee*, 4 May 2020, vsee.com/what-is-telemedicine/.

xviii Lougheed T. (2019). Time to embrace the promise of virtual health care. *CMAJ : Canadian Medical Association journal = journal de l'Association medicale canadienne*, 191(11), E320–E321. https://doi.org/10.1503/cmaj.109-5720

xix Wicklund, E. (2020, April 14). *Coronavirus Gives People a Reason to Use Telehealth, But Doubts Remain*. mHealthIntelligence. https://mhealthintelligence.com/news/coronavirus-gives-people-a-reason-to-use-telehealth-but-doubts-remain.

xx E. Klecun-Dabrowska, T. C., RL. Bashshur, T. G. R., D. Hailey, A. O., PJ. Hu, P. Y. C., R. Currell, C. U., PA. Jennett, L. A. H., ...

R. Whittemore, S. K. C. (1970, January 1). *Implementing telehealth to support medical practice in rural/remote regions: what are the conditions for success?* Implementation Science. https://link.springer.com/article/10.1186/1748-5908-1-18.

xxi Chipidza, F. E., Wallwork, R. S., & Stern, T. A. (2015). Impact of the Doctor-Patient Relationship. *The primary care companion for CNS disorders*, 17(5), 10.4088/PCC.15f01840. https://doi.org/10.4088/PCC.15f01840

xxii Agarwal, A. K., & Murinson, B. B. (2012). New dimensions in patient-
physician interaction: values, autonomy, and medical
information in the patient-centered clinical
encounter. *Rambam Maimonides medical journal*, 3(3), e0017.
https://doi.org/10.5041/RMMJ.10085

xxiii R. Kaba, P. Sooriakumaran, The evolution of the doctor-patient relationship, International Journal of Surgery, Volume 5, Issue 1, 2007, Pages 57-65, ISSN 1743-9191, https://doi.org/10.1016/j.ijsu.2006.01.005.

xxiv Office, S. (2016, April 4). *Cypress*. 5 Patient Benefits of Concierge Medicine. https://www.yourcypress.com/news/april-2016/patient-benefits.

xxv Choi, N.G., Choi, B.Y., DiNitto, D.M. *et al*. Fall-related emergency department visits and hospitalizations among community-dwelling older adults: examination of health problems and injury characteristics. *BMC Geriatr* **19**, 303 (2019). https://doi.org/10.1186/s12877-019-1329-2

xxvi (2020). *Resources For Finding A Lab*. Lab Tests Online. https://labtestsonline.org/resources-finding-lab

xxvii Office, S. (2016, April 4). *Cypress.* 5 Patient Benefits of Concierge Medicine. https://www.yourcypress.com/news/april-2016/patient-benefits.

xxviii Finlan, T. (Ed.). (2020, January). *Occupational Therapy (for Parents) - Nemours KidsHealth.* KidsHealth. https://kidshealth.org/en/parents/occupational-therapy.html.

xxix Lyon, OTR/L, S. (2020, June 5). *Telehealth Occupational Therapy Guide - OT Potential.* Telehealth Occupational Therapy Guide. https://otpotential.com/blog/telehealth-occupational-therapy.

xxx "Caregivers Taking Care of Themselves." *Cancer.Net*, 10 Dec. 2020, www.cancer.net/coping-with-cancer/caring-loved-one/caregivers-taking-care-themselves.

xxxi The Mind Tools Content Team. *How to Juggle Caregiving Responsibilities and Work: Keeping it Together When Work and Care Commitments are Pulling You Apart.* The Mind Tools Content Team Publishers https://www.mindtools.com/pages/article/juggling-career-and-care.htm.

xxxii Sullivan, A. B., & Miller, D. (2015). Who is Taking Care of the Caregiver?. *Journal of patient experience,* 2(1), 7–12. https://doi.org/10.1177/237437431500200103

xxxiii Forducey, P. G., Glueckauf, R. L., Bergquist, T. F., Maheu, M. M., & Yutsis, M. (2012). Telehealth for persons with severe functional disabilities and their caregivers: facilitating self-care management in the home setting. *Psychological services,* 9(2), 144–162. https://doi.org/10.1037/a0028112

xxxiv National Institute of Mental Health, S. (2015). *Chronic Illness & Mental Health*. National Institute of Mental Health. https://www.nimh.nih.gov/health/publications/chronic-illness-mental-health/index.shtml.

xxxv Bresnick, J. (2016, July 8). Why Mental Healthcare is Key to Population Health Management. https://healthitanalytics.com/news/why-mental-healthcare-is-key-to-population-health-management.

xxxvi Chong, J., Neurology, D. of, And, Moreno, F., Psychiatry, D. of, Legha, R. K., ... Moreno., J. C. and F. (2012, May 7). Feasibility and Acceptability of Clinic-Based Telepsychiatry for Low-Income Hispanic Primary Care Patients. https://www.liebertpub.com/doi/abs/10.1089/tmj.2011.0126.

xxxvii Rosenblatt, R. A., & Hart, L. G. (2000). Physicians and rural America. *The Western journal of medicine, 173*(5), 348–351. https://doi.org/10.1136/ewjm.173.5.348

xxxviii Potyraj, J. (2016, February 11). *The Quality of US Healthcare Compared With the World*. AJMC. https://www.ajmc.com/view/the-quality-of-us-healthcare-compared-with-the-world.

xxxix Ryan P. (2009). Integrated Theory of Health Behavior Change: background and intervention development. *Clinical nurse specialist CNS, 23*(3), 161–172. https://doi.org/10.1097/NUR.0b013e3181a42373

xl Krupinski, E. A., & Bernard, J. (2014). Standards and Guidelines in Telemedicine and Telehealth. Healthcare (Basel, Switzerland), 2(1), 74–93. https://doi.org/10.3390/healthcare2010074

xli N/A. *What is Mental Health Parity?* NAMI: What is Mental Health Parity? https://www.nami.org/Your-Journey/Individuals-with-Mental-Illness/Understanding-Health-Insurance/What-is-Mental-Health-Parity.

xlii Martina, D. (2019). Advance Care Planning among Healthcare Professionals in Asia: A Systematic Review of Knowledge, Attitude and Experience. https://doi.org/10.26226/morressier.5c76c8b3e2ea5a7237611 f95

xliii Crowley, R., Daniel, H., Cooney, T. G., Engel, L. S., Gantzer, H. E., Erickson, S. M., ... Burstin, H. (2020, October 13). *Envisioning a Better U.S. Health Care System for All: Coverage and Cost of Care.* Annals of Internal Medicine. https://www.acpjournals.org/doi/full/10.7326/M19-2415.

xliv Staff. (2018, May 30). *American Health Care: Health Spending and the Federal Budget.* Committee for a Responsible Federal Budget. https://www.crfb.org/papers/american-health-care-health-spending-and-federal-budget.

xlv N/A. "5 Approved Doctor Notes: Edit & Download." *Hloom.com*, 17 Apr. 2019, www.hloom.com/resources/templates/more/doctors-note.

xlvi Becker, T. D., Lin, H. C., & Miller, V. A. (2018). A pilot study of observed physician-parent-child communication and child satisfaction in a gastroenterology clinic. *Patient preference and*

adherence, *12,*   1327–1335.
https://doi.org/10.2147/PPA.S171620

xlvii Pomey, M. P., Ghadiri, D. P., Karazivan, P., Fernandez, N., & Clavel, N. (2015). Patients as partners: a qualitative study of patients' engagement in their health care. *PloS one, 10*(4), e0122499. https://doi.org/10.1371/journal.pone.0122499

xlviii Esposito, L., & Khan, A. (2019, December 18). *13 Questions Your Doctor Wants You to Ask.* 13 Questions Doctors Wish Their Patients   Would   Ask. https://health.usnews.com/conditions/slideshows/questi ons-doctors-wish-their-patients-would-ask?slide=15.

xlix Mathioudakis, A., Rousalova, I., Gagnat, A. A., Saad, N., & Hardavella, G. (2016). How to keep good clinical records. *Breathe   (Sheffield,   England), 12*(4),   369–373. https://doi.org/10.1183/20734735.018016

l Becker, T. D., Lin, H. C., & Miller, V. A. (2018). A pilot study of observed physician-parent-child communication and child satisfaction in a gastroenterology clinic. *Patient preference and adherence, 12,*   1327–1335. https://doi.org/10.2147/PPA.S171620

li Staff (2020). *Fever: Symptoms, Causes, Care & Treatment.* Cleveland Clinic. https://my.clevelandclinic.org/health/symptoms/10880-fever.

lii Pomey, M. P., Ghadiri, D. P., Karazivan, P., Fernandez, N., & Clavel, N. (2015). Patients as partners: a qualitative study of patients' engagement in their health care. *PloS one, 10*(4), e0122499. https://doi.org/10.1371/journal.pone.0122499

liii McCracken MD, G. (2015, April 15). 9 Myths of Telemedicine. https://blog.evisit.com/virtual-care-blog/9-myths-of-telemedicine.

liv Paavola, A. (2018, March 1). *Fact or fiction: Top 6 telehealth myths to know. The number of health systems adopting telehealth programs is on pace to double in the next few years as a result of the shift to consumer-driven healthcare, which has been expedited by policy changes and technology advancements.* Fact or fiction: Top 6 telehealth myths to know. https://www.beckershospitalreview.com/telehealth/fact-or-fiction-top-6-telehealth-myths-to-know.html.

lv Well, A. (2017, February 10). The top five myths of telehealth. https://www.healthcareitnews.com/sponsored-content/top-five-myths-telehealth.

lvi Herman, B. (2016, February 20). *Virtual reality: More insurers are embracing telehealth.* Modern Healthcare. https://www.modernhealthcare.com/article/20160220/MAGAZINE/302209980/virtual-reality-more-insurers-are-embracing-telehealth.

lvii Dinesen, B., Nonnecke, B., Lindeman, D., Toft, E., Kidholm, K., Jethwani, K., Young, H. M., Spindler, H., Oestergaard, C. U., Southard, J. A., Gutierrez, M., Anderson, N., Albert, N. M., Han, J. J., & Nesbitt, T. (2016). Personalized Telehealth in the Future: A Global Research Agenda. *Journal of medical Internet research*, 18(3), e53. https://doi.org/10.2196/jmir.5257

lviii Slight, S. P., Berner, E. S., Galanter, W., Huff, S., Lambert, B. L., Lannon, C., Lehmann, C. U., McCourt, B. J., McNamara, M., Menachemi, N., Payne, T. H., Spooner, S. A., Schiff, G. D., Wang, T. Y., Akincigil, A., Crystal, S., Fortmann, S. P., & Bates, D. W. (2015). Meaningful Use of Electronic Health

Records: Experiences From the Field and Future Opportunities. *JMIR medical informatics, 3*(3), e30. https://doi.org/10.2196/medinform.4457

lix Beach, M. C., Inui, T., & Relationship-Centered Care Research Network (2006). Relationship-centered care. A constructive reframing. *Journal of general internal medicine, 21 Suppl 1*(Suppl 1), S3–S8. https://doi.org/10.1111/j.1525-1497.2006.00302.x